NUTRITION
DIAB

Penelope S. ‗‗‗‗‗, ‗‗‗‗., ‗.‗., ‗.‗.‗.
Charlotte S. Harker, Ph.D., R.D.
Catherine E. Higgins, M.S., R.D., C.D.E.
Marvin C. Mengel, M.D.

SOME ADVANCE REVIEWS

This is a comprehensive review of the multiple approaches to nutrition care for the patient with diabetes mellitus. Dr. Easton et al. have presented nutritional care for the diabetic patient from infants to the elderly in a well-balanced and detailed forum. The book is well indexed and the outline is easy to follow. I would consider this book to have a well-deserved place in the library of all members on the health care team for the patient with diabetes mellitus.

Sanford N. Plevin, M.D.
Director
Mease Diabetes Treatment Center

An excellent reference for new or experienced dietitians involved in education of people with diabetes mellitus. It encourages dietitians to be nonjudgmental and realistic in their expectations of clients' learning and compliance abilities and to foster this attitude in the clients they teach. The glossary of terms is excellent and could serve as a valued resource alone.

Michele W. Keane, Ph.D., R.D., L.D.
Assistant Professor, Department of Dietetics and Nutrition
Florida International University

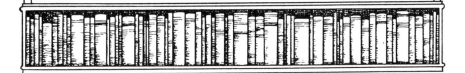

Nutrition Care of People with Diabetes Mellitus

A Nutrition Reference for Health Professionals

Nutrition Care
of People
with Diabetes Mellitus
A Nutrition Reference
for Health Professionals

Penelope S. Easton, Ph.D., R.D., C.D.E.
Charlotte S. Harker, Ph.D., R.D.
Catherine E. Higgins, M.S., R.D., C.D.E.
Marvin C. Mengel, M.D.

Food Products Press
New York • London • Sydney

Published by

Food Products Press, 10 Alice Street, Binghamton, NY 13904-1580
EUROSPAN/Food Products Press, 3 Henrietta Street, London. WC2E 8LU England
ASTAM/Haworth, 162-168 Parramatta Road, Stanmore (Sydney), N.S.W. 2048 Australia

Food Products Press is a subsidiary of The Haworth Press, Inc., 10 Alice Street, Binghamton,
NY 13904-1580.

Library of Congress Cataloging-in-Publication Data

Nutrition care of people with diabetes mellitus : a nutrition reference for health professionals
/ Penelope S. Easton ... [et al.].
   p. cm.
Includes bibliographical references.
Includes index.
ISBN 1-56022-004-X (alk paper) — ISBN 1-56022-007-4 (alk. paper softcover)
1. Diabetes—Diet therapy. 2. Diabetes—Nutritional aspects. I. Easton, Penelope S.
[DNLM: 1. Diabetic Diet. WK 818 N97616]
RC662.N87 1990
616.4'620654—dc20
DNLM/DLC
for Library of Congress
90-13936
CIP

CONTENTS

List of Tables

ABOUT THE AUTHORS

Penelope S. Easton, Ph.D., R.D., C.D.E., now retired from 24 years of experience in teaching dietetics and nutrition at Florida International University (Miami) and Indiana State University (Terre Haute), now lives in Zephyrhills, Florida. She taught patients for four years as an army dietitian and three years as a public health nutritionist, in Alaska and Florida, as well as four years as a hospital dietitian in small hospitals. She has concentrated on the problems in nutrition education for the treatment of diabetes mellitus for the past twelve years. She is a certified diabetes educator and is particularly concerned with the problems of elderly people.

Charlotte S. Harker, Ph.D., R.D., is a professor emerita after 25 years of college teaching in nutrition and dietetics at Indiana State University. She developed curriculum and prepared educational programs and materials for all levels of learning. Her primary responsibilities were for the educational and clinical preparation of dietitians. She now is in private practice in Indiana as a Nutrition Consultant.

Catherine E. Higgins, M.S., R.D., C.D.E., has been a diabetes educator, hospital dietitian, and school food service supervisor. She is currently Chief Clinical Dietitian, Singing River Hospital, Pascagoula, Mississippi.

Marvin C. Mengel, M.D., is an endocrinologist in private practice in Orlando, Florida, and Director of the Diabetes Treatment Center at Orlando Regional Medical Center. He has been medical director or responsible for both in-patient and out-patient diabetes education programs. He is a graduate of Johns Hopkins University School of Medicine where he did his fellowship training in Internal Medicine and Endocrinology. He is currently on the faculties of the University of Florida and the University of Central Florida.

Preface

This book has been written to provide general practitioners of medicine, nursing and dietetics with comprehensive up-to-date nutrition advice related to diabetes mellitus. This vital aspect of treatment, nutrition, often has not received sufficient attention and the lack of success in food intake management may influence the whole course of the disease. The principal goal of this book is to provide health care providers with treatment strategies which encourage as many patients as possible to approach appropriate blood glucose levels while living their normal lives.

The authors have noted that many of their patients have achieved good control in spite of, rather than because of, dietary advice which did not fit their needs. The strategies and concern in this book are designed to help the patient achieve control more quickly than the trial and error method so many have used. Practical strategies keep them within the medical care system. Other patients have a need for a different plan, a new approach, a way to start or start over. This book has many ideas for health professionals to use or adapt.

The book is written with the assumption that the users will have a basic knowledge of diabetes and traditional treatment regimens. Recommendations are given only for treatment that is directly related to or greatly influenced by food intake. Other medical recommendations are not included because many references are available on these aspects.

We have used numerous references as well as many of our experiences in treating and teaching patients. We have worked to give the most up-to-date information and theories with some evaluations and predictions of their successes. Reference material has been cited when the information is controversial or involves new research and ideas.

This book is divided into six sections. The first section outlines the different competency levels and traditional instruction strategies and alternatives. The following two sections are devoted to consideration of the early years and the adult and aging years. Sections IV and V emphasize specialized conditions and weight correction. Section VI covers more detailed information about food components and nutritional guidelines. The use of computerized nutrient analysis is addressed where appropriate. A comprehensive glossary of nutrition terms relating to diabetes is included.

Editorial Note: Since the trend appears to be to return to traditional terms for the most common types of diabetes mellitus, insulin dependent (IDDM) and non-insulin dependent (NIDDM) have been used primarily. Readers are reminded that IDDM is also called Type I and NIDDM, Type II.

Acknowledgements

Sincere appreciation is extended to the Diabetes Care Center, Humana Hospital-Lucerne, Orlando, Florida for sponsoring the initial prototype of the handbook.

Acknowledgement is made to the original panel of 46 dietitians, 32 nurses, 28 physicians who responded to the needs survey. A special thank you is extended to all of our patients and co-workers for the useful ideas and experiences they have shared with us.

Special acknowledgement is made to Sara Blackburn, D.Sc., R.D.; Vivian L. Witkoff, M.S., R.D.; Lois Allen Busone, M.S., R.D.; John Malone, M.D.; Cheryl Scott, R.N. and Mary B. Somers, M.S., R.D.

All the authors are grateful to Linda Ammon, M.S., R.D. for her work with the patients using the Food Choice Plan and her contributions as one of the authors of the prototype handbook.

Section I:
Diet Instruction Competencies

INTRODUCTION

Lists of competencies for dietetic management have been included to assist those health professionals working in health departments, clinics and offices where the client is seen infrequently or only for a short visit to pick up insulin or other prescription items. Minimal competencies are designed for individual counseling from medical personnel although, realistically, these sessions might be conducted by a medical aide or even clinical clerical personnel or volunteers. Trained personnel are considered to be preferable for instruction but at a minimal competency level they may be able to only review the records. Learner and adequacy level competencies require more highly trained medical personnel and frequent follow up. Group instruction may possibly be useful, for some instruction beyond the minimal level but it is confusing for introduction to care.

Minimal Level

These competencies are absolutely minimal competencies. They should be taught and monitored constantly to determine changes in needs and attitudes, and to respond to alterations in treatment regimens. It is possible that at this level the care giver may need the education as well or in lieu of education of the patient. Although mastery of minimal competencies cannot guarantee adherence to and improvement in disease control, it is safe to assume that few patients can achieve adequate control without these competencies. Materials should be in the patient's primary language with drawings and pictures that cover *only* the competencies of this level.

Although there are materials available in languages such as Spanish, these usually are far too complicated for this level. The language may be different from that spoken by the client and the foods may be unfamiliar as well. For example, people of Mexican and Cuban backgrounds have very different food habits and language patterns.

Counselors should be realistic in giving advice. If the client eats only one-dish meals such as stew or refried beans, then the size of serving and the amount of fat added should be discussed rather than an attempt made for a "well-balanced" diet.

Learner Level

This level assumes that minimal skills are learned although repeated reviews of all skills are indicated. For example, long time use of serving sizes may change from the prescribed plan. A 1/2 cup measure may easily creep up to 3/4 cup, a teaspoon of salad dressing may become a tablespoon.

Attention to nutritional adequacy is introduced at this level and some simple food pattern for nutrient adequacy is advised. Some plans such as the Basic Four Food Groups or Healthy Food Choices (see Section VI, Table 27) may be used if these foods are found to be available in the client's lifestyle.

Additional materials to those at the Minimal Level should be included and written in the patient's primary language with line drawings and/or pictures. Patients with special conditions such as pregnancy or accompanying illness must reach this level if the prevention of complications is to be achieved.

Adequacy Level

This level requires use of the whole health care team and constant monitoring of the blood levels is necessary. Ability to understand and demonstrate competency at this level does not assure adherence nor does it guarantee control. If the client understands his/her own disease state and his individual problems, group sessions or support groups concerning food may be useful.

SECTION I: CHAPTER I
DIET INSTRUCTION COMPETENCIES
FOR NON-OBESE PERSON WITH DIABETES

Minimal Level

I. Objectives

    A. Approach euglycemia.
    B. Prevent life threatening episodes.

II. Patient Competencies

    A. Plan a daily schedule of actual food items, not lists. This should include only foods available to and liked by client.
    B. Know appropriate foods for emergencies such as hypoglycemia or illness.

III. Specific Instruction

    A. Demonstrate reasonable food intake divided into 4 to 6 meals.
    B. Show serving sizes:

        1. Level measurement of teaspoons, tablespoons, 1/2 cup, and 1 cup and differences with heaping or rounded measurements.
        2. Three ounce portion of meats and amount of fat used in preparation or left on meat.
        3. Compositions of mixed dishes—sources of "hidden" fat and sugar.

    C. Show that no foods, with possible exception of lettuce, other greens, and celery, can be eaten in unlimited amounts and then the dressing or other fats must be considered.
    D. Show 3 to 4 caloric equivalents for each meal, also one or two options for illness/emergencies.
    E. Demonstrate foods to eat to prevent severe hypoglycemia. Show how to change meal times or amounts if hypoglycemia occurs frequently or persists.
    F. Have two conferences with a counselor on a one-to-one basis.

1. First conference

    a. Choose foods likely to be eaten during day.
    b. Show serving sizes for each of these.
    c. Give emergency information.
    d. Hand out written materials explaining above in patient's primary language and use drawings and pictures as well in case literacy is limited.

2. Second conference

    a. Evaluate knowledge from first conference.
    b. Give additional information on caloric equivalents and menu changes for activities.
    c. Emphasize serving sizes, food preparation, and purchasing techniques.

G. Demonstration materials needed include:

1. Household measuring tools/supplies (ex: teaspoon; tablespoon; coffee cup; 4 oz, 8 oz and 12 oz glasses; measuring cups.)
2. Food models especially those showing 3 oz portions of meats and foods commonly used such as fast foods. (Do not use complicated lists of foods such as Exchange Lists.)

Learner Level

I. Objectives

A. Approach euglycemia.
B. Prevent life threatening episodes.
C. Promote good nutrition.

II. Patient Competencies

A. Minimal techniques mastered.
B. Know adaptations for changes in schedule, exercise, weight, age, growth, other disorders, and personal and health considerations.
C. Know where to find reference material for additional substitutions or specific needs.

D. Know about sweeteners and specialized foods.
E. Know some food patterns such as Basic Four Food Groups to aid in reaching good nutritional status.

III. Specific Instruction, 2 to 3 sessions after minimal competency is reached.

A. Revise food schedule to allow for changes.
B. Know how to substitute new foods that are more desirable than presently used foods.
C. Know how to adapt food preparation techniques and allow for foods prepared out of the home.
D. Know low caloric foods to use and those to avoid.
E. Know where to find valid information.
F. Develop some call back or reinforcement schedule.

IV. Demonstration Materials

A. Household measuring tools/supplies.
B. Food models.
C. Food labels.
D. Charts of caloric values of foods.
E. Healthy Food Choices and/or Four Food Group materials.

Adequacy Level

I. Objectives

A. Maintenance of acceptable blood glucose level with life changes and stresses.
B. Recognition of desirable diet changes including need for additional instruction.
C. Ability to evaluate new treatments, diets, and dietary aids in terms of effectiveness and desirability.
D. Ability to recognize frauds and fads.
E. Techniques developed to control disorder within desired social, physical, and personal aspects of life.

II. Patient Competencies

A. Learner level techniques mastered.
B. Know adaptations for lifestyle changes.

    C. Have current reference materials and knowledge of current resources and support groups available.

    D. Demonstrate ability to monitor disease and prevent and/or control emergencies.

III. Specific Instruction

    A. Review competencies.

    B. Demonstrate adaptation of meal plans.

    C. Participate in group meetings and/or membership in local support groups.

    D. Provide library of information pamphlets and alternate food patterns.

    E. Demonstration materials needed include:

        1. Blood glucose determination kits.

        2. Pamphlets on food plans.

        3. Reference materials and information about support groups.

SECTION I: CHAPTER II
DIET INSTRUCTION COMPETENCIES
FOR OBESE PERSON WITH DIABETES

Minimal Level

I. Objectives

    A. Approach euglycemia.

    B. Approach weight correction.

II. Patient Competencies

    A. Plan daily schedule of food which has a maximum of 4 meals a day spaced at least 4 to 5 hours apart.

    B. Know serving sizes for foods.

    C. Know food preparation and dilution techniques.

III. Specific Instruction

    A. Demonstrate reasonable food intake divided into 3 to 4 meals. Use actual foods in client's lifestyle.

B. Demonstrate serving sizes.
C. Show that no food can be eaten in unlimited amounts.
D. Show that a smaller serving of any food has a lower caloric value than a larger serving of the same food.
E. Demonstrate how cooking in or adding fat can double or triple caloric contribution.
F. Demonstrate how to cut away visible fat and avoid or severely limit serving sizes of high fat/high sugar foods.
G. Establish realistic weight goals and plan for enough weight loss to effect blood glucose.
H. Show how food can be "diluted" by cellulose or water. (Examples: salads and broth soups.)
I. Show how dressings, gravies, fats, and sugars that are not visible can increase the caloric density of a food.

IV. Demonstration materials

A. Household measuring tools/supplies.
B. Food models or actual foods that are in client's lifestyle.
C. Materials in client's language; use line drawings and pictures.

Learner Level

I. Objectives

A. Approach euglycemia.
B. Approach and maintain acceptable body weight.
C. Promote good nutrition.
D. Maintain minimal level competencies to help prevent complications.

II. Patient competencies

A. Minimal techniques mastered.
B. Appropriate evaluation of weight correction progress.
C. Know where to find reference material for additional substitutes or specific needs.
D. Develop 2 to 3 behavior modification techniques to encourage progress.

E. Establish network, peer groups and/or periodic record-keep-ing to improve weight correction or control.

F. Know food patterns such as Basic Four Food Groups, or Healthy Food Choices to aid in reaching good nutritional status.

G. Be familiar with blood lipid levels and associated cardiovas-cular disease risks.

H. Promote reasonable increases in energy utilization by in-creasing walking or other exercise and decreasing sitting or sleeping.

I. Promote non-food related social activities.

J. Suggest such behavior techniques as:

1. Eat from smaller plates.
2. Dilute foods with water or fiber and discourage use of fat in preparation.
3. Decrease fat and sugar consumption, including sugars from fruits and juices.
4. Increase milk, especially skim milk.
5. Learn to reward self with non-food rewards.
6. Be aware of food fads and frauds.

III. Specific Instruction

A. Demonstrate reasonable food intake divided into 3 to 4 meals.

B. Demonstrate serving sizes — for example, quantities in dif-ferent sized glasses/cups.

C. Show that no food can be eaten in unlimited amounts.

D. Show that a small sized serving of any food has fewer calo-ries than a larger serving.

E. Demonstrate how cooking in or adding fat can double or triple caloric contribution.

F. Demonstrate how to cut away visible fat and how to avoid or severely limit serving sizes of high fat/high sugar foods.

G. Help establish realistic weight goals and scheduled losses.

H. Show how food can be "diluted" by cellulose or water. (Example: salads and broth soups.)

I. Show how dressings, gravies, fats and sugar that are not evident can increase the caloric density of a food.

IV. Demonstration materials

    A. Household measures and utensils.
    B. Food models or actual foods.
    C. Drawings and pictures.

Adequacy Level

I. Objectives

    A. Maintenance of acceptable blood glucose level with life changes and stresses.
    B. Recognition of changes including need for additional instruction.
    C. Ability to evaluate new treatments, diets, and dietary aids in terms of effectiveness and desirability.
    D. Ability to recognize frauds and fads.
    E. Development of techniques to control disorder within desired social, physical, and personal aspects of life.
    F. Ability to vary food and patterns to prevent boredom.

II. Patient Competencies

    A. Master minimal and learner techniques.
    B. Ability to evaluate weight correction progress.
    C. Knowledge of appropriate sources of information for specific needs.
    D. Ability to develop and implement additional behavior modification techniques.
    E. Establish network, support groups and/or record-keeping to improve weight correction and control.
    F. Knowledge of a variety of food patterns.
    G. Implement reasonable increase in energy use.

III. Specific Instruction

    A. Revise competencies and make necessary adaptation of meal plans or menus.

    B. Participate in group meetings. Membership in local support groups.

    C. Obtain library of information pamphlets and alternate food patterns.

IV. Demonstration materials

    A. Blood glucose determination kits.

    B. Pamphlets on food plans. Exchange Lists may be used at this level if desired.

    C. Reference materials and information about support groups.

SECTION I: CHAPTER III
THE DIET PRESCRIPTION
FOR AMBULATORY PATIENTS (ENERGY)

Determining the energy* aspect of a diet prescription is more difficult than usually considered. The authors recommend a diet prescription based on present body weight and estimated energy use (Table 1). There is good evidence that total body weight correlates with energy use[1] and hence it is important to base an energy prescription on actual weight rather than an "ideal" or "desirable" weight.

The energy (caloric) prescription should be in accord with the client's lifestyle, both present and past. It should involve few calculations and be monitored and revised on a regular basis.

The Harker/Easton Estimate (Table 1) is easy to use. It involves one clinical judgment and one calculation using present body weight in pounds. The Harker/Easton system is based on the RDA's[2] and the work of Durnin and Passmore.[3] The reliability of the easy to use Harker/Easton Method to estimate energy use was compared to the adjusted Harris Benedict formula in 132 subjects.[4,5]

Both methods gave similar results for women. Values for men in the 23-50, and 51-70 age groups were slightly higher in Harker/Easton than with the Harris-Benedict adjusted formula.

---

*Authors' Note: This book uses the terminology energy (kcal) to indicate the potential energy contribution of food and energy use by the body. (See glossary for calories and kcals.)

TABLE 1. Harker/Easton Estimation of Energy Use Ranges of Values

Activity Factors

Males Age	Inactive Obese kcals/lb	Light Activity Normal kcals/lb	Very Active Thin kcals/lb
15-18	16 to 18	19 to 21	22 to 24
19-22	14 to 16	17 to 21	20 to 22
23-50	12 to 14	15 to 17	18 to 20
51-70	11 to 12	14 to 15	16 to 17
70+	9 to 10	11 to 12	13 to 14
Females Age			
15-18	13 to 15	16 to 18	19 to 21
19-22	11 to 13	14 to 16	17 to 19
23-50	10 to 12	13 to 15	16 to 18
51-70	9 to 10	11 to 12	13 to 14
70+	8 to 9	10 to 11	12 to 13

The study of the Harker/Easton method was based upon the following definitions:

Weight: Classes based on 1983 Metropolitan Height/Weight Tables (Appendix I)

Obese: 10% or more of highest value in large frame category
Thin: 10% or more of lowest value in small frame category

Usual Daily Activity Levels:

Inactive: Individuals not meeting any of the following criteria

Light Activity: 2 hours or less in level IV activity or 1 hour or less in level V activity

Moderate Activity: 4 hours or more in level IV activity or 2 hours of more in level V activity

Very Active: 6 hours or more in level IV activity or
                      3 hours of more in level V activity

Activity Classification (Appendix II):

Level I: Sitting — using minimum muscles such as eating,
Sedentary   studying, knitting, office work, playing cards.

Level II: Some standing and walking, some large muscle
Very Light   work — driving car, ironing, laboratory work, walking
                slowly, personal necessities.

Level III: Primarily standing, some movement of large mus-
Light   cles — cooking, doing dishes (hand), hand laundry,
                walking normally, expert golfer.

Level IV: Standing with movement of large muscles — walking
Moderate   downstairs, cleaning vigorously, gardening, walking
                very rapidly, playing volleyball, golfing, washing
                car.

Level V: Primarily large muscles used strenuously — bicycling,
Heavy   dancing (vigorously), gymnastics, swimming, run-
                ning, playing tennis, walking upstairs.

Both the Harker/Easton and Harris-Benedict systems were based on normal individuals so the effects of diabetes, if any, are not known.

The amount of adjustment of energy use either for the addition needed for weight gain or subtraction for weight loss should be carefully chosen. The 500 kcal usually used may be too high for a person using 1200 kcal a day and too little for a person using 2500 kcal a day.

The caloric deficit should not be punitive nor based on the assumption that the patient will "cheat." Some people do not adhere to prescriptions by eating more, others by eating far less. Diet instruction is a necessary aspect for the understanding of the energy prescription.

As the body weight changes, the energy use will change as well. This change may partly explain the weight loss plateaus although adaptation to starvation may be a factor also. After 20% weight loss, the prescription should be recalculated. When people with IDDM receive enough insulin to control blood glucose, weight will be gained or regained. Unwelcome weight gain should be monitored carefully and a revised prescription given. A form useful for calculating the energy prescription is given in Table 2.

After the energy prescription is determined, the food should be spaced during the day according to the patient's activities, blood sugar swings such as the dawn phenomenon,[6] and types and amounts of blood sugar lowering medications. This should be done with the cooperation of all health team members as well as the patient. The proportioning of food according to percentage of energy nutrients is discussed in following chapters.

SECTION I: CHAPTER IV
INSTRUCTION SYSTEMS FOR DIABETES MELLITUS;
DIET INSTRUCTION GOALS AND METHODS

Sufficient evidence is available to show that no instruction method assures adherence. All instruction methods depend on the needs and comprehension of the client and the skills and resources of the teacher.

Instruction for following a diet to treat diabetes is further complicated by the myths, beliefs, and misinformation that abound in the media and folklore.

Recommendations and considerations for diet instruction are found in all sections of this book, but the commonly used systems, plans and techniques are described and evaluated in the sections following the goals for dietary treatment.

Goals for Dietary Treatment

The "Nutritional Recommendations and Principles for Individuals with Diabetes Mellitus: 1986"[7] is the basis for the following discussion. The authors have identified and commented on specific parts and aspects of the published goals.

TABLE 2. Form for Calculating Energy Prescription

Energy prescription for _____
                         Name of Patient

1. Present weight in pounds _____

2. Activity factor _____ from Table 1[*]
    for sex, age, and activity/weight classification.

3. Estimation of present energy use:

    _____ X _____ = _____ kcal/day
    Present wt.   Factor from
    in pounds   Table 1.
    (1. above)   (2. above)

4. Adjustment for weight gain or loss
    +/- _____ kcal/day

5. Energy prescription   _____ kcal/day

6. Special conditions and limitations:

[*] The use of height/weight tables and precise energy
level categories are necessary only for research or
very precise calculations. An estimate by a clinical
dietitian, exercise physiologist or physician is all
that is usually required.

1. Approach, achieve and maintain euglycemia.
   Comment: This goal, if achieved, will often accomplish some
   of the ancillary goals. Priority ranking of goals is essential and
   multiple restrictions should be minimized or avoided unless
   there is acute physiological justification. Most newly diagnosed
   patients need an absolute minimum of restrictions although occasionally a patient is anxious to avoid as many problems as
   possible and will want all recommended restrictions.
2. Achieve acceptable lipid levels.
   Comment: This is listed as a second goal here, although it is
   included as part of goal one of the A.D.A. list.[7] Sometimes the
   achievement of normal euglycemia will result in acceptable
   lipid levels. In other circumstances the dietary adjustments
   necessary for goal one are enough for the patient to compre-
   hend initially. It may be goal one, however, in patients in a
   high risk category.

3. Maintain normal growth rate for children and adolescents.

   Comment: Again this is goal one for specific age groups. The balance between insulin and food needed for growth is delicate and needs constant attention and revision.

4. Provide adequate nutrition for the pregnant woman, the fetus, and lactation.

   Comment: The special need during pregnancy makes this the first goal for pregnant women with diabetes or gestational diabetes to ensure a healthy baby.

5. Establish schedules in the timing of meals and snacks to prevent inordinate swings in blood glucose levels for people using exogenous insulin.

   Comment: The use of self glucose monitoring allows for the adjustment of insulin; however, the adjustment of food must be addressed to prevent excess weight gain.

6. Determine meal plans appropriate for the individual's lifestyle.

   Comment: It is necessary to take into consideration the patient's constant daily changes in lifestyle and teach dietary manipulation for these.

7. Teach obese patients to manage their weight.

   Comment: Weight correction and control strategies need constant supervision, support and updating.

8. Improve overall health of people with diabetes.

   Comment: The usual restrictions for management of diabetes by diet encourage the use of nutrient dense foods. This goal should not be expressed or imposed on the non-interested patient at the beginning of treatment.

Food and Nutrition Recommendations

In this discussion the goals listed previously are being considered in relation to the recommendations of the Diabetes Association's Task Force on Nutrition 1988.[8] The recommendations are given in reference to the 1980 RDAs.[9]

While all recommendations should be considered, the instruction for the patient should be determined by treatment priorities, and the patient's lifestyle. Each recommendation below is reviewed by the authors in terms of the usual priority it should be given and comments are made concerning feasibility of attainment.

Energy (kcals)

Calories should be prescribed to achieve and maintain a desirable body weight.

Comment: The term desirable body weight (see Glossary and Appendix I) has very different meanings to medical personnel, caregivers and patients. Often it is calculated as the so-called Ideal Body Weight estimation (Appendix I) or taken from the 1959 or 1983 Metropolitan Weight/Height Charts. This weight may seem alarmingly low and completely unobtainable to the obese person with NIDDM and outrageously high to the thin person with IDDM. The authors recommend use of estimated present use (Table 1) and adaptation necessary with attainable and acceptable goals for the patient. The goal weight listed on the chart and given to patients should be time and situation driven. Example: X lb (gain/loss) by Y (date).

Carbohydrate Intake

The amount of carbohydrates should be liberalized, ideally up to 55-60% of the total kilocalories, and individualized, with the amount dependent on the impact on blood glucose and lipid levels and individual eating patterns.

Comment: High intakes should be achieved gradually for patients who have had very different diets previously. There is some evidence that people needing large amounts of food (4000-6000 kcals) may find this impossible (see athletics and exercise) and there is some evidence that it may increase insulin needs. Patients with NIDDM may experience elevated triglycerides.[10]

Whenever acceptable to the patient, foods containing unrefined carbohydrate with fiber should be substituted for highly refined carbohydrates, which are low in fiber.

Comment: The role of fiber and high fiber diets are discussed in Section VI. The social consequences of high fiber foods and the effects of different kinds of fiber as well as the malabsorption of some minerals in high fiber diets make this a recommendation requiring restraint, especially for the very young and sometimes the very old.

> In some individuals, modest amounts of sucrose and other refined sugars may be acceptable, contingent on metabolic control and body weight.

Comment: Clinicians have long noted that many patients can handle reasonable amounts of sucrose without deleterious effects. Dietary experts have also been aware that sucrose is present in fruits and other common foods (see Section VI, Chapter V). The concerns about sucrose as with other foods is the amount taken and the spacing. This recommendation is encouraging in terms of truth in instruction even if it is viewed with alarm by some and may lead to problems in some patients.[10,11]

Protein Intake

> Americans in general consume too much protein. The recommended dietary allowance (RDA) for protein is 0.8 g/kg of body weight for adults. Elderly subjects may require more than the RDA. There are circumstances where the protein intake may be reduced, e.g., in patients with incipient renal disease.

Comment: Much education is needed for specific groups regarding protein. Comments concerning this are to be found in appropriate sections. It is important to note here that up to 1/2 of protein can be converted to glucose and that neuropathy occurs in 1/5-1/3 of people with diabetes mellitus within 15 years of onset. Protein intake based on body weight may not be satisfactory for obese patients because it would be too high. The often used figures of protein intake as 15-20% of total caloric intake may be low for very low caloric diets and too high for people with high energy needs. A clinical judgement of grams of protein which includes consideration of the quality of protein eaten is needed for each patient. For high caloric/high carbohydrate diets an unrealistic protein value may be obtained with the 3 gram protein value for a cereal/bread exchange. Using actual values for breads used instead of exchange value may be better.

Alternative Sweeteners

The use of various nutritive and non-nutritive sweeteners is acceptable in the management of diabetes.

Comment: Sweeteners including sucrose are discussed in the Glossary and Section VI, Chapter V. Cautions concerning these are included under pregnancy (Section II, Chapter V).

Salt Intake

Many Americans eat more salt (NaCL) than is necessary. The recommended sodium intake is 1000 mg/1000 kcal not to exceed 3000 mg/day. In some hypertensive subjects, salt may be harmful, and therefore intake should be reduced. Severe sodium restriction could also be harmful for certain individuals with poorly controlled diabetes, postural hypotension, and fluid imbalance.

Comment: Salt intake is discussed in several sections of this book (Athletics and Exercise, Other Disease Conditions and the Elderly). For the initial diet prescription without complicating conditions it becomes a secondary goal. A lowered intake of food automatically lowers salt intake. This may be restriction enough for many.

Alcohol

The same cautions regarding the use of alcohol that apply to the general public apply to people with diabetes. Specific problems may occur with hypoglycemia, neuropathy, glycemic control, obesity, and/or hyperlipidemia.

Comment: The use of alcoholic beverages should be discussed with most patients. The energy contribution of alcoholic beverages and the interaction of alcohol with medications must be considered.

Total Fat and Cholesterol

Total fat and cholesterol intake should be restricted. Total fat should comprise < 30% of total calories and cholesterol < 300 mg/day.

Comment: This recommendation and its accompanying comments concerning the difficulty of compliance are endorsed by the authors in view of the relative incompleteness of research. Fat controlled diets are discussed in Section IV, Chapter V. The recommendation of less than 30% of dietary caloric intake as fat may be very difficult to achieve on high caloric diets or with people who are used to and like a high fat diet.

Vitamins and Minerals

Vitamins and minerals should meet the recommended requirement for health.

Comment: There is no evidence of extra need for vitamins and minerals by patients with diabetes except in cases of diagnosed deficiencies. The Surgeon General's Report on Nutrition and Health[12] states that most Americans generally do not need nutrient supplements and that there are no known benefits to healthy people consuming excess amounts. The excess amounts can be harmful.

Techniques Used to Determine Usual Diet Intake

Food Records

The use of a food record from one to seven days duration is a commonly employed effort to estimate usual food intake. Often a new patient is asked to bring such a record to the first visit. This may or may not be a true record of what was eaten for the time specified but does alert the patient to food habits and serving sizes. Forms suggested for this use are in Appendix III. If a food record is submitted, it *must* be reviewed at the visit where it is presented or the food record loses its effectiveness.

Advantages:

1. Patient starts to study foods and amounts.
2. Foods commonly used by patient may be evident.
3. May serve as a basis of instruction.

Disadvantages:

1. Patients may find this threatening and time consuming.
2. Health provider may assume the one record is typical and will rate it "good" or "bad."
3. Computer analysis may give false sense of accuracy, adequacy and deficiencies.

Food Recall

A food recall (usually for 24 hours) is even more frequently used by dietitians than a record. The form used for the record can be given to the patient as a recall form or a system of instructions and probing questions can be used by health personnel. Health personnel should be aware that guilt, and inaccurate measures and faulty recall may make this a less than perfect system. The recall is useful to determine ethnic food patterns and meal times.

In the hands of skillful interviewers these methods are useful and can double as a teaching technique. The authors recommend some alternate systems such as the Food Choice Plan to save time and allow the patient to "start over" when interview time is limited. A good recall cannot be completed in less than thirty (30) minutes and it is more important for the patient to focus on future behavior patterns than past.

Advantages:

1. A good interviewer can establish rapport and find out a great deal about a person's lifestyle.

2. Recalling by time of day and willingness to note unusual circumstances is possible and will encourage responses.
3. The patient may start to think of food timing, choices, and amounts.

Disadvantages:

1. The patient may try to please and report what the interviewer wants to hear.
2. Patients may not understand language, descriptions, or names of food, or may be unfamiliar with weights and measures.
3. Reported food may be modified by patient because of guilt or to protect food provider. (This is especially true when children are asked to report intakes.)

"24 Hour Recall" Probe Items and Suggestions:

Sample Probe Items: (Sometimes obtaining an activity record simultaneously is useful and less threatening.)

A. It is useful in planning your menus to know what, how much, and when you eat in a day. Please tell me what you ate (or what you did) in the last 24 hours (or yesterday).
B. What is the first thing you ate or drank (or what time did you get up—what did you do first) in the morning?
   Note: All answers should be accepted without judgment! Everyone has some information about what should or should not be eaten. A nonjudgmental attitude may help to establish communication.
C. What was the first thing you ate/drank in the past 24 hours? Do not say "what did you eat for breakfast?" Use such questions as "was that all? Did you have anything on your cereal? How were your eggs cooked? How big was the cup/glass/bowl? How full was the spoon/cup/bowl?"
D. When did you eat or drink anything again? Use questions such as "how big was the slice? How thick? Did you put anything on the vegetables?", etc.
E. When the recall is used for planning a diet for a person with diabetes, the following questions should be asked:

1. Is this your usual meal pattern?
2. How many times a week do you eat like this?
3. What are the difficulties?
4. What habits are you able to change?
5. What foods are very important to you?

Food Frequency

A food frequency inventory which asks how many times a week/month a person eats a food may be helpful in research or food distribution programs. It is nearly impossible to use these as an indication of nutrient intake except for one or two nutrients.

Because of the current interest in cholesterol and saturated fats a form to estimate intakes of these foods by a food frequency is included in Appendix III. The authors do not think that actual intake in terms of grams/milligrams can be determined using this method but they have devised a scoring system to estimate degrees of intake.

Computerized analysis of food frequencies for individuals does not appear to be worth the cost or time necessary to do this and implies a degree of accuracy not possible to determine.

Group Instruction and Feelings About Diets

The authors have found that group meetings for diet instruction are fraught with dangers. Few people understand their own prescriptions and disease state well enough to choose relevant information. A strong group participant may negate the health team members' information.

Group instruction limited to such topics as serving sizes, caloric value of foods, cutting down food intake may be useful.

An information test is often useful in instructing groups although some people find this threatening. In Appendix V an information test the authors have given to groups of both patients and professionals is shown. Also included is a sample detailed answer sheet which is useful in reinforcing learning and is essential to clarify the items because a "yes" or "no" answer is insufficient.

A sample attitude survey is included (Appendix V) which may be useful in detecting how patients feel about their diets. The survey may be as useful for the patient as for the instructor because it helps the patient examine feelings about the diet which may be general feelings about the disease. Since decisions about food are constant, the feelings of the person who must make these decisions may be important.

Cost of Dietary Advice

Cost of various types of diabetic dietary programs cannot be determined here in dollars, but the actual number of hours of education involved is of concern and can be from 6 to 12 hours or more for assessing and educating a patient on the diabetic diet.[13]

SECTION I: CHAPTER V
TEACHING TECHNIQUES AND STRATEGIES

Diet Counselor

The personal charactcristics of a diet counselor are probably far less important than the counselor's knowledge, attitude, and teaching skills. Since health personnel come from the general public, it is reasonable to assume that they may represent all kinds of people, fat, thin, old, young, ill, or well. It is unreasonable for them to be burdened with a "be perfect" commandment. Patients, especially obese ones with diabetes are very sensitive and guilt-ridden. Patients are quick to note if the health team member views them with rejection or repugnance because of their size, age, race, economic status, or lack of control.

Factors to Consider in Choosing Diet Instruction Techniques

A. Choose techniques that are appropriate for instructional level (see this section under "Diet Instruction Competencies for Non-Obese Person with Diabetes" and "Diet Instruction Competencies for Obese Person with Diabetes"), literacy level, patient's lifestyle, type of disease and control, and patient's interest in dietary adherence.
B. Consider cost of materials and if any particular foods are advised.
C. Rank multiple restrictions in order of priority according to patient's condition and interest (ex: a person at high risk for car-

diovascular disease (CVD) may need to have fat restrictions first, or one with a renal risk have protein restrictions first).
  D. Be willing to adapt current techniques or to try a new system that replaces one that the patient dislikes.
  E. Be aware that no system is accurate or best in all instances.

Diet Instruction Techniques

A. Weighed Foods: Used in conjunction with other systems.

Advantages:

1. Alerts person to serving sizes and importance of controlling amounts of foods.

Disadvantages:

1. Is tedious and may encourage compulsive behavior.
2. Does not guarantee accuracy because fat weighs less than water and proteins. Food that has less water such as dried bread or toast will weigh less.

B. Measured Foods: Important at beginning for people who are unfamiliar with serving sizes.

Disadvantages:

1. Inaccuracies with dilution may occur.

C. Exchange Lists

The most commonly used food sort system was devised by members of the American Diabetes Association and The American Dietetic Association in 1950. The most recent revision (1986) contains some important changes from the 1976 lists.[14] The differences in values are listed in Table 3.

Advantages:

1. Useful as a quick calculation tool and teaching method of food choices.
2. The universality of use makes the system an attractive one for patients who are comfortable with it.

TABLE 3. Comparison of Nutritional Values per Serving of the 1986 and 1976 A.D.A. Exchange Lists

Food Group	1986				1976			
	CHO	Prot	Fat	Energy	CHO	Prot	Fat	Energy
	<--grams-->			kcal	<--grams-->			kcal
Starch/Bread	15	3	-	80	15	2	-	70
Meat/Meat Substitutes								
Lean	-	7	3	55	-	7	3	55
Med. fat	-	7	5	75	-	7	5.5	77.5
High fat	-	7	8	100	-	7	8	100
Vegetables	5	2	-	25	5	2	-	25
Fruits	15	-	-	60	10	-	-	40
Milk								
Skim	12	8	-	90	12	8	-	80
Lowfat	12	8	5	120	12	8	5	120
Whole	12	8	8	150	12	8	8	150
Fat	-	-	5	45	-	-	5	45

3. Many materials, cookbooks and publications use exchange lists.
4. The new version includes combination foods and allows for occasional foods.
5. Some food service establishments have food exchange lists for their products (i.e., McDonalds).
6. High fiber foods (3 or more grams per serving) are marked with a wheat emblem. The high sodium foods (400 mg or more of sodium per serving) are marked with a salt shaker.
7. A distinction is made between high fat, medium fat, and lean meats and between whole, lowfat and very lowfat milk.

Disadvantages:

1. The complexity of the system is not easily mastered by all patients and has led to the development of other systems.[15,16,17]
2. The values do not "add up" according to the usual system of 4 kcal/gm of carbohydrate and 4 kcal/gm for protein and 9 kcal/

gm of fat. In some cases this is due to the traces of fat in the foods or small amounts of protein.

3. A variety of measuring systems are used: ounces, pounds, cups, tablespoons, teaspoons, grams and kilograms.
4. The six lists have a total of 325 items, each with its own serving size given, which makes for constant referral to the lists a necessity for all patients until they become used to the amounts. This may be discouraging for many.
5. The differences in actual food nutrients and these grouped nutrients may be important if a person uses many servings of a particular food and certainly needs to be examined closely in terms of using them in research studies.
6. Some values appear to be low in comparison to the nutritional level of the product, e.g., yogurt.
7. Some commercial products and computerized programs list exchanges for a product although that exchange does not exist in the food, e.g., Weight Watchers German Chocolate Cake lists one fruit exchange on the label although the product contains no fruit.
8. Many materials using the older values still exist which may confuse a patient until all materials are updated. The new values increased the calculated caloric values for most diets from 13-16% but of course did not change the actual values in foods.

A comprehensive booklet on Exchange Lists is available from the American Diabetes Association and The American Dietetic Association.[14] (Members of the The American Dietetic Association receive a professional discount.)

D. Food Choice Plan (FCP)

The authors of this book developed and tested a system called the Food Choice Plan in the early 1980s.[17] This is a system of serving size control and record keeping; no food is forbidden. The goal of the Food Choice Plan is to approach euglycemia and to postpone sophisticated dietary considerations until the patient has good understanding of this primary goal.

Patients choose actual foods for menus for three days. The energy prescriptions and serving sizes are then checked by a dietitian and the patient's written menus become a food contract. The approved menus are duplicated to use for daily records and patients are asked to return records at appropriate intervals. Alternate foods eaten are recorded and guilt about such choices is minimized. Frequent alternates indicate the need for new menus or additional choices. (FCP protocol and forms are in the Appendix IV.)

Advantages:

1. The patient has planned for actual food intake, times, and amounts. Three alternate foods are usually determined and a comment section for substitutions is provided.
2. The duplication of the menu sheet when used for a record cuts down on the number of items that must be recorded (foods are just circled).
3. The system requires that a patient and dietitian have face to face discussion of food, not an away-from-the-patient review of a history or recall by the dietitian. Follow-up is required.
4. The menus become a contract and additional restrictions can easily be incorporated. Negotiation is encouraged.

Disadvantages:

1. Some patients are not ready or are unwilling to plan menus or keep records.
2. Some dietitians are unable to devote the initial two hours (usually in one hour segments) and several follow-up visits.
3. FCP is best as an initial ambulatory menu and record keeping rarely continues after two to four weeks.
4. The "permissiveness" of the system alarms some patients and health professionals.
5. Teaching serving sizes and caloric contributions of foods in lifestyle is essential and may not be done by staff.

E. Healthy Food Choices

Shortly following the publication of the 1986 Exchange Lists, the committee which developed them published a large poster sized pamphlet which follows the dietary guidelines. This colorful easy to use pamphlet is reasonably priced and is available from The American Dietetic Association. A simplified 16 page version entitled "Eating Healthy Foods" by the American Diabetes Association and The American Dietetic Association, 1988, is available from The American Dietetic Association, Chicago.

Advantages:

1. The alternative lists are called choices not exchanges and are short lists.
2. It can be easily adopted for alternate lifestyles, languages and limited literacy.
3. A menu form is given and additional ones available.
4. It encourages use of ordinary foods and family eating patterns.

Disadvantages:

1. The pamphlet is multi-purpose and therefore does not use the term diabetes, which some patients may find troublesome.
2. It may be confusing for in-hospital use but is good for discharge teaching.

F. Calorie Counting

Used in many programs. With this approach, a broad range of foods is included. Calories are totaled at the end of each day and should approximate the calorie prescription.

Kilocalories may be divided among different food groups in order to meet nutritional considerations. A dietitian teaches the importance of good nutrition and how it affects diabetes.

Some references of caloric counts and a suitable form are useful. Some computerized programs do this electronically. Follow-up of records is usually necessary.[15]

G. Point System

Instead of counting kilocalories, point systems have been devised. Meals can be calculated by points to adjust for insulin.[17] Computer programs utilizing the point systems are available for home computers. The programs keep track of the number of points used and help adjust the meal plan for illness or special occasions.

H. Personal Guidelines

The Kentucky Diabetes Foundation[15] developed a system of this type. These diets emphasize foods that are high in complex carbohydrates and fiber, and low in fat. A dietitian teaches how to select foods wisely. For instance, skim or lowfat milk is recommended instead of whole milk. Guidelines are given to the patient gradually. Certain foods are limited but none is totally eliminated.

With the help of a dietitian, the number of food servings and the size of food portions for each meal are planned. The serving sizes vary and the portion sizes serve as guidelines.

I. Total Available Glucose (TAG) (17):

This system is based on the concept that the three major nutrients (carbohydrate, protein, and fat) ultimately break down into glucose. The nutrients are given values — carbohydrate 100%; protein 58%; fat 19%. These values are applied to the Exchange System for meal planning. For example, a bread exchange has 16.8 TAG, meat 4.6 and fruit 15. The main emphasis is to adjust and regulate insulin.

J. High Carbohydrate-High Fiber (HCF)

These are are food lists and individualized calculations emphasizing fiber and were developed by the University of Kentucky group.

K. So-Called ADA Diets

Some years ago the ADA published some allotments of food exchanges at different caloric category levels. These were merely suggestions and not officially endorsed schedules. They were so widely used and published by some drug companies, hospital diet manuals and weight control groups that they became known as A.D.A. diets. *There are no A.D.A. diets* and diet orders should read: IDDM Diet of ____kcal or NIDDM diet of ____kcal. Any lipid, sodium or special meal size or times should be added. (See Diet Rx, this section, under ''The Diet Prescription for Ambulatory Patients).

These old patterns almost always included a meat (egg) at breakfast and often several servings of fruit. Such foods at breakfast are undesirable for many patients. Since some patterns may be necessary for hospitals and nursing homes, patterns for 1000-1200 kcal and 1500-1700 kcal and 2000-2200 kcal are given in Appendix VI. Higher caloric patterns need to be carefully planned for the individual even in the hospital.

Editorial Note: Although some references have listed a "set point diet," the authors have reservations about promising patients that they can achieve a "set point" that will take the place of conscious control. They think it is possible that people who are obese and/or who have diabetes may not have a developed set point mechanism if one exists. If such mechanisms exist in these people, they may be so high that an acceptable weight is unreachable.

REFERENCES

1. Forbes, G.B.: Energy need for weight maintenance in human beings: Effect of body size and composition. J Am Diet Assoc 89: 4:499, Apr 1989.

2. Food and Nutrition Board, National Research Council: Recommended Dietary Allowances, 7th revised ed.: Washington, D.C., National Academy of Sciences, 1968.

3. Durnin, J.V.G.A. and Passmore, R.: Energy, Work and Leisure, London: Heineman Educational Books, Ltd., 1967.

4. Harris, J.A., Benedict, F.G.: A Biometric Study of Basal Metabolism in Man: Carnegie Institute of Washington, 1919.

5. Hensler, C., Easton, P.S., Harker, C.S., Johnson, P.M.: Comparison of methods to estimate energy use. Suppl J. Am Diet Assoc 89:9:A107, Sep 1989.

6. Stephenson, J.M., and Schernthaner, G.: Dawn phenomenon and somozyi effect in IDDM. Diabetes Care 12:4:245, Apr 1989.

7. American Diabetes Association: Position Paper, Nutritional recommendations and principles for individuals with diabetes mellitus: 1986. Diabetes Care 10:1:126, Jan/Feb 1987.

8. American Diabetes Association: Report of the American Diabetes Task Force on Nutrition. Diabetes Care 11:2:127, Feb 1988.

9. Food and Nutrition Board, National Research Council. Recommended Dietary Allowances, 9th revised ed.: Washington, D.C., National Academy of Sciences 1980.

10. Hollenbeck, C., Coulston, A.M., Reaven, G.M.: Effects of sucrose on carbohydrate and lipid metabolism in NIDDM patients. Diabetes Care 12:1:62, Jan 1989.

11. Abraira, C., and Derler, J.: Large variations of sucrose in constant carbohydrate diets in Type II diabetes. Am J Med 84:193 Feb 1988.

12. The Surgeon General's Report on Nutrition and Health, U.S. Department of Health and Human Services, DHHS (PHS) Publication No. 88-50210, Washington, D.C. 1988.

13. Disbrow, D.D., Costs and benefits of nutrition services: A literature review. Suppl J Amer Diet Assoc 89:4, Apr 1989.

14. American Diabetes Association, American Dietetic Association Exchange Lists for Meal Planning. Revised 1986: The American Dietetic Association, Chicago, 1986.

15. Gershberg, H.: Office care of newly diagnosed IDDM. Diabetes Care, 11:4:294, Apr 1988.

16. Welon, N., Homoko, C., Petit, W.: Office care of newly diagnosed IDDM. Diabetes Care, 12:1:40, Jan 1989.

17. Diabetes Care and Education Practice Group: Meal Planning Approaches in the Nutrition Management of the Person with Diabetes. The American Dietetic Association, Chicago, 1987.

Section II:
Nutrition in the Early Years

INTRODUCTION

Since the treatment of the infant born to a woman with diabetes is under the care of the attending pediatrician and since the occurrence of diabetes in infancy and early childhood is rare, the authors wish to emphasize that the nutritional treatment should be supervised by a specialist in diabetes. The information given here is for infants and children in general. There is a great "need for research on the safety and efficiency of dietary restrictions in childhood."[1]

SECTION II: CHAPTER I
INFANCY

The greatest difficulty in feeding the infant with diabetes is adjusting the insulin to handle actual intake and changing needs for growth and activity. Sometimes, although glycemic control is achieved, insufficient food is given for growth and development resulting in growth retardation or actual stunting. Neurological impairment may occur coincidentally with inadequate nutrition.

Ordinarily, infant formulas contribute 20-40 kcal per ounce. If dilution is not accurately determined or the infant does not swallow all of the formula or regurgitates it, the intake can vary from recommended intake. Insulin adjustments are needed.

Weight, height, and head circumference changes do show growth and help estimate growth rates. The infant with diabetes should have growth grids kept accurately and regularly. Growth grids will not help determine day-to-day food management; therefore, glucose monitoring is a good recommendation. Formula adjustment is probably needed at least monthly.

The addition of foods other than formula is open to many questions. The primary source of energy for the child up to six months is infant formula. The addition of a source of ascorbic acid and probably iron may be necessary before 6 months. (Iron needs can be met with three tablespoons of rice cereal.) At six months foods can be introduced. The later time for introducing solid foods appears to prevent allergies and postpone or prevent obesity. Solid foods introduced early do not appear to cut down on night feedings. *Caution*: Nibbles of food and bites of food from caretakers should be discouraged for the child with diabetes because of the difficulty in estimating content and amount as well as sanitary conditions.

Caution: Low fat or skim milk is not advised even for obese infants because of the child's inability to handle large solute loads. There appears to be a need to have cholesterol in the diet of infants. Table 4 shows some conditions affecting food intake of infants.

Although lists showing energy nutrient equivalents (Exchange Lists) are available for baby foods, they are of little use. Charts listing kilocalories may be a better guide. Caregivers should be cautioned against combination foods such as casseroles, desserts, and soups. The ideal foods to be introduced after cereals (with no sugar added) are vegetables; although realistically fruits are preferred by the infant. Serving sizes of fruits especially should be watched. Fruit puddings are not recommended because these contribute sugars and carbohydrates mainly and only limited amounts of vitamins and minerals. Although the recommended intakes are met initially by formula, some idea of the amount of food an infant or young

TABLE 4. Conditions Affecting Food Intake

Condition	Occurrence	Remedy	Caution
Dehydration	Common in an infant	Only water should be given unless severely malnourished	Mixtures with electrolytes are recommended. Caloric intake of liquids should be considered.
Fever	Frequent	Increase in formula 1-2 oz/feeding.	Body tempererature increases of 1° F, increases BMR 7%.
Regurgitation and vomiting	Common	Food replacement may be needed.	Frequent projectile vomiting should be reported immediately.

child needs is useful. The pattern below indicates how the recommended allowances can be met.

Foods

Foods which will supply the recommended dietary allowance for energy for 1 day are:[2]

A. 2-6 months	28-32 oz. human milk or infant formula (95-145 kcal/kg)(43-67 kcal/lb)
B. 6-10 months	30-38 oz. human milk or infant formula 1-3 small servings daily of foods listed below. (80-135 kcal/kg)(30-36 kcal/lb)
C. 10-12 months	24 oz. milk or infant formula (1000 kcal) plus: 2 (1/2 cup) servings of strained vegetables; 1/2 cup infant cereal (dry, dilute with some milk); 1 slice of bread or 6 crackers; 1/3 cup junior meats; 1 cup of juice or fresh fruit (such as bananas, pears, peaches)

The infant with IDDM should have a regular schedule for food according to activity and sleep patterns.

SECTION II: CHAPTER II
CHILDREN – 1 TO 10 YEARS

General Description

The use of too little insulin or insufficient food is a real danger in treating children. The misconception that the amount of insulin determines the severity of the disease may be a contributing factor to the growth retardation which has occurred from insufficient food intake in children.

The advent of home glucose monitoring has allowed a great deal of freedom and helped parents and children alike understand how to control blood glucose. However, high energy intake when adequately supplied with insulin may lead to obesity. The amounts and kinds of food are important for the child with diabetes. A child's dietary prescription should be checked at least every two months with attention to growth, appetite, food likes, and changes in energy use.

If the child does not drink fluid milk, the best sources of the nutrients in milk are yogurt and cheeses. The plain yogurts have 150 kilocalories per cup and the sweetened ones have 240-260 kilocalories because of added sugars! Children with very high energy needs (ex. 2000 kcal) may need the higher caloric foods. Most cheeses are high in fat and sodium. Milk can be used in cooking or even low caloric puddings may be used. A lactase deficiency usually does not occur before 8 years so fluid milk is advised if at all possible. Low fat chocolate milk is a possibility if milk is merely disliked. If breads and cereals are substituted for disliked vegetables, not only the carbohydrate content but also the decreased amounts of ascorbic acid and folic acid should be considered. Potatoes are a good source of ascorbic acid and should not be forbidden, but should not be given as chips, and only rarely as French fries. Sauces, butters, and fats used in preparation or as an accompaniment to vegetables must be considered, especially if enough are used to calculate as additional kilocalories.

Serving sizes of meals and the ways in which all foods are prepared are very important. A child's plate in a restaurant is usually approximately a 2-3 oz. entree portion and not an adult serving size. This should be considered in calculating the diet pattern.

Food Schedules

The child, one to five years, may need to have several schedules planned. Rarely does a child have a simple schedule which is useful seven days a week. The beginning hour will probably change on parents' leisure and recreation days. Efforts to make schedules too rigid may induce stress in the child, siblings, and/or caregivers.

Various strategies are available which allow the child to live a life compatible with his peers. Children can learn food substitutes such as those in caloric charts. For example, 1/2 cup of ice cream might be used in place of a slice of bread with 2 teaspoons of peanut butter. The use of caloric equivalents is usually satisfactory and does not seem to upset the blood glucose unless the caloric equivalents are all from sugars. (See Kilocalorie Chart in Appendix XI.)

Determining energy needs and expenditure for different activities and the fear of hypoglycemia are real problems. The amount of energy used is often overestimated; therefore, hyperglycemia may result. The blood glucose does decrease with exercise in children who are well controlled but insulin cannot be omitted. Regularly scheduled exercise should be worked into the diet/insulin regimen. Caution: Vigorous exercise should not be prohibited and slow increases in exercise level and timing with glucose monitoring are advised. (See Exercise & Athletics.)

Even very young children are aware of society's emphasis on obesity. Eating disorders can begin early. Table 5 gives recommendations for diet planning for children with IDDM and Table 6 the recommended energy intakes for children of various ages.

Food for Children at School

Most public schools in America have a feeding program for children. Some of these employ dietitians, but all make an effort to accommodate children with special needs such as those with diabetes if at all possible. However, the responsibility for food choices must be that of the child. Children who expect food substitutions and then choose foods not traditionally allowed for people with diabetes will receive little sympathy. Food substitutions that are unusual often cause school personnel great distress and confusion. School food service personnel cannot legally or ethically allow the child different treatment unless appropriate prescriptions are on file.

In view of the importance of foods with adequate nutrients, if at all possible the basic school lunch menu as served should be used. Adjustments can be made in other meals. However, school breakfasts may not be a good choice if the child has morning hyperglycemia, takes a long bus ride, or the breakfast hour is too close to lunch.

It is important that children from low income families have their insulin planned to take advantage of the breakfast for the quality of nutrients provided if sufficient food is not available at home. (See Table 8.)

There are several alternatives depending on the needs of the child and the parent: (1) checking the published school menu and helping

TABLE 5. Recommendations for Diet Planning for Children with IDDM

Recommendation	Advantages	Caution
1. Children with diabetes need planned meals and snacks	Consideration should be given to intermittent snacking as a way of life for Americans. Calculation of nutrient intake as snacks and scheduling insulin is advised.	Uncontrolled "nibbling" may occur unless snacks are planned and monitored.
2. Have whole family follow the diet.	Sound nutrition is the goal of any diet prescribed for treatment of diabetes and these diets are usually appropriate for all people.	May make child resented by siblings.
3. Weigh/measure all foods.	Useful at first, especially meats. Teaches serving sizes.	Is cumbersome and food composition differs greatly by preparation method and dilution by water and/or fiber.
4. Remove sugars candy, etc. from environment.	Allows child to manage foods easier.	Does not teach serving sizes and may perpetuate myth that sugar is "poison".

the child plan what to eat and how much of each food; (2) packing a lunch to fit the food pattern planned; (3) packing alternative items for those the child will not or should not eat. For example: planning to eat one half of a brownie, (large with frosting 192 kcal) is a rather difficult situation for some children and an alternative plan which would be appropriate might be to omit the dessert if one is offered, or carry a lower caloric dessert such as one chocolate chip cookie (approximately 100 kcal).

Children should carry some source of readily available glucose. For example, glucose tablets. They should also be aware that too frequent use of these indicates poor control and a check up is needed. Teachers and other children need to learn about diabetes. The newly diagnosed child may need support and help in this. Glucose monitoring at school is possible and under ideal conditions can be a learning experience for teachers, parents, and students alike. (See hypoglycemic treatment later in this chapter.)

The trend in diabetes management today is moving toward

TABLE 6. Recommended Energy Intakes for Children*

Age (years)		Average kcal/lb body weight	Median Weights and Heights (lb)	(in)
Infants	0.0-0.5	49	13	24
	0.5-1.0	45	20	28
Children	1-3	46	29	35
	4-6	41	44	44
	7-10	32	62	52
Males	11-14	25	99	62
	15-18	20	145	69
Females	11-14	21	101	62
	15-18	18	120	64

* NRC-NAS: Recommended Dietary Allowances. 1989 (3).

The energy allowances given in the table are proposed as averages and approximate allowances for feeding groups of children. More appropriate allowances for individual children can be obtained from observations of growth, activity, appetite and weight gain in relation to the deposits of body fat. For the child with diabetes mellitus the body weight should be carefully monitored and a balance between the amount of insulin and the food intake maintained. A satisfactory growth rate and body weight depends upon both the amount of insulin and the food intake.

achieving a more normal lifestyle for the child with diabetes rather than adhering to traditional ideas such as no sugar or "fruit only" for desserts. However, since some school personnel, even nurses, may not have received current information about a diabetic diet, management problems may arise. For example, an oatmeal cookie may be allowed for the child although the school personnel may think that is inappropriate. The substitutions and food choices dictated by serving size systems now recommended seem radical to teachers and school personnel. The most useful control may be class scheduling and, if possible, physical education should occur after lunch rather than a snack being given before or too soon after the activity. Variable lunch hours make control more difficult, but a regular lunch hour should not be required at the expense of belonging to the peer group.

If the child feels "different" or is not allowed to be with friends or classmates because of lunch hours, a snack may be a better alternative so that physical education can be allowed before lunch. Some children prefer not to be labeled "Diabetic" and want their problem told to the teacher and school nurse only. The symptoms of hypoglycemia should be taught to teachers and other school administrators.

The following school meals are given to show common patterns. The caloric content may be adapted by substituting low fat milk and/or omitting bread/butter or desserts (Tables 7 and 8).

School lunch regulations require that 1/3 of the R.D.A.s for a child be met at the lunch. No such recommendation is made for breakfast but a pattern of foods is listed. This pattern allows choices of either bread, cereals, or meats and therefore the child with diabetes needs a somewhat flexible breakfast menu.

SECTION II: CHAPTER III
ADOLESCENCE

The push toward the achievement and maintenance of euglycemia is needed due to the relationship of metabolic control to normal growth and development and the apparent prevention or postponement of the development of chronic complications. The monitoring of the adolescent with IDDM requires that they have a caregiver and healthcare supervisor who understand the physical needs and psychological change and pressures during adolescence.

In recent years the carbohydrate component of the diet has been increased because this has been shown to improve glycemic control. Treatment strategies of multiple injections, insulin pumps, and home glucose monitoring have liberalized meal scheduling. Not only is a high carbohydrate diet more acceptable to adolescents but also improvement in health appears to occur.

Current recommendations for nutrient distribution are given in Section I, Chapter III. The fat recommendation may be low for the active adolescent. To eat 2500-4000 kcal with only 83 to 133 grams of fat is difficult because it involves so much food by weight. Such food patterns are different from those of the usual active adolescent. Therefore, this goal may need to be postponed or modified until control is achieved and lifestyle changes unless there is a very elevated blood cholesterol or family history of early heart attacks. Table 9 gives dietary recommendations for adolescents.

In planning the diet with the adolescent, habits, preferences and activity should be considered. The estimated caloric intake should be divided into three meals and one or more snacks so that adequate food is consumed at each meal to prevent hypoglycemia. Emphasis

TABLE 7. Energy Estimates of Some School Food Service Meals

	Amount	Total Energy (kcal)	Protein (gm)	Carbo-hydrate (gm)
Menu I				
Pizza	1 piece	236	12.00	28.30
Tossed Salad	3 leaves	6.5	.45	1.50
Celery	1/2 stalk	4	.20	1.00
Tomatoes	1 slice	3	1.00	.45
Green Pepper	1 piece	2	.12	.48
Salad Dressing	1 Tbsp.	57	.08	2.40
Apple-sauce	1/4 cup	58	.25	15.00
Oatmeal Cookie	1	63	.90	10.30
Milk	1/2 pint	159	8.50	12.00
Total		589	23.50	71.43
Menu II				
Sloppy Joe	1/3 cup	245	15.08	8.75
Bun	1	89	2.50	15.90
Cabbage Slaw	1/4 cup	45	.60	3.50
Corn	1/4 cup	35	1.10	8.20
Potato Chips	1/2 oz	81	.76	7.10
Brownie/ Icing	1	159	8.50	12.00
Butter	1 tsp.	36	.05	-
Total		690	28.59	55.45

TABLE 7 (continued)

	Amount	Total Energy (kcal)	Protein (gm)	Carbo-hydrate (gm)
Menu III				
Roast				
Turkey	2 oz	80	12.40	-
Salad-				
Potato	1/2 cup	94	2.10	12.30
Peas	1/4 cup	29	2.25	4.70
Roll	1	113	3.10	20.10
Butter	1 tsp	36	.05	-
Peanut				
Butter				
Cookie	1 piece	166	3.24	24.70
Milk	1/2 pint	159	8.50	12.00
Total		677	31.64	73.80

These values are calculated from Bowes and Church's Food Values of Portions Commonly Used for school recipes and portion sizes served. J. Wynn, unpublished research 1983.

should be placed on maintaining a consistent food intake by following a basic meal schedule. The inclusion of popular and familiar foods is recommended to promote compliance to the dietary regimen. Thus, foods totally restricted are very few; however, serving sizes should be monitored. The adolescent needs to know how to adapt for unusual situations.

Numerous meal plans are available to assist in developing the basic meal plan as discussed in Section I, Chapter III. Adjustments of energy intake should be made periodically to maintain weight and to provide for normal growth and development. Vitamin and mineral requirements are the same for children whether or not they have diabetes.

Special precautions should be taken when choosing/performing an activity. It is generally suggested that when the blood glucose is 200 mg/day or above and ketones are in the urine, exercise should be avoided. (Note: The exact glucose level to be used varies according to different authorities and the physician in charge should deter-

TABLE 8. Average Nutrient Contributions of Hillsborough County School Meals*

	Lunch Elementary	Lunch High School	Breakfast Elementary
Total kcals	700	870	335
Total protein (gm)	28	34	12
Protein % of kcal	15	15	14
Carbohydrate % of kcal	50	46	50
Fat % of kcal	35	39	36
Vitamin A % of RDA	80[1]	80[2]	16[1]
Vitamin C % of RDA	70[1]	70[2]	30[1]
Calcium % of RDA	60[1]	40[2]	40[1]
Iron % of RDA	40[1]	30[2]	15[1]

[1] RDA used was for children 7 - 10 (1980)
[2] RDA used was for boys 15 - 18 (1980)

* Warch, B., Easton, P., Somers, M., 1989

mine this for each person.) At such times exercise may even result in an increase in blood glucose.

Parties or other special occasions may increase food consumption which can be offset by increased activity or insulin. With home glucose monitoring, additional insulin such as regular insulin, under a physician's guidelines, may be given to offset the increased food intake. The use of alcoholic beverages must be considered and appropriate cautions and amounts discussed.

Eating Disorders

Young people often feel compelled to achieve and maintain a weight which is far below an ideal weight for height. Comments by friends or relatives about the need to lose weight may lead to obsessive weight restriction behaviors in which energy intake is greatly decreased and energy expenditure is increased.

Some adolescents having diabetes with these goals will not restrict food intake but will decrease insulin, the end result being the same: low body weight. This leads to extremely poor control and could become a serious ketotic condition. The misuses of insulin to accomplish low body weights really amounts to bulimia. The authors have called this bulimia of diabetes (glossary) although they have never seen the term used elsewhere.

The extent of eating disorders has not been adequately studied but the health professional should watch for symptoms. Weight gain following diagnosis and establishment of control should be explained and monitored. The fear of hypoglycemia and use of glucose monitoring techniques can lead to excess food intake.

The use of judgmental terms such as "good," "healthy," or "junk" foods is inappropriate and may invite undesired behaviors.

The stresses of adolescence appear to be the same for those with IDDM as for other teenagers but the consequences of irregular habits and stress mean that management of food intake and glucose balance should be appropriately addressed by clinical personnel.[4]

The weight gain found to accompany tight glycemic control must be avoided to prevent eating disorders and onset of obesity.

The establishment of energy needs for activity, growth and maturation must be carefully balanced with insulin used. This should be done non-judgmentally and frequently. The need to increase insulin to control hyperglycemia should be carefully watched to see if the long term need is really to decrease food.[4]

SECTION II: CHAPTER IV
PHYSICAL EXERCISE AND ATHLETICS

Physical activity (exercise) is a vital component of the treatment regimen both for weight loss and control as well as obtaining improved glucose control. The benefits of exercise, both physical and psychological, are well documented and individuals with diabetes obtain the same benefits as the person without diabetes. An exercise prescription should be developed with the individual just as with any other treatment plan. The importance of nutrition during athletic events is currently being emphasized. More attention is needed during training and when more than usual physical activity occurs.

Athletes are constantly exposed to nutritional myths and misinformation. Winning is often attributed to some magic potion or ritual rather than talent or training. Some of these "magical" potions may be harmful for the person with diabetes. Some nutritional misconceptions of athletes are shown in Table 10.

Blood glucose monitoring is strongly recommended especially for the IDDM patient. During exercise glycogen from muscle and liver storage is depleted. After exercise these stores are replenished. Thus, the effect of exercise on diabetes control can last from 24 to 48 hours. Post exercise late onset (PEL) hypoglycemia may occur for 6-15 hours following strenuous exercise and have few warning signals (PEL hypoglycemia).[5] Improved plasma glucose with decreased insulin needs is often noted. In fact, after a strenuous activity such as singles tennis, hypoglycemic episodes may occur more frequently. This may be a result of lower blood glucose levels as well as failure to adjust insulin dosage. Prevention of PEL hypogly-

TABLE 9. Dietary Recommendations for Adolescents

Recommendation(s)	Approach(es)
1. Observe energy nutrient distribution for carbohydrate (50-60%), protein (15-20%), fat (30%)	(a) Liberalization may be indicated for adolescent eating 2 or more meals away from home. (b) Instruction on basic principles. (c) Instruction on obvious sources of fat.
2. Adequate protein intake for growth/development	(a) Protein recommendations are for 1 gm/kg ages 11-14 decreasing to 0.8 gm/kg at age 19 for males, age 15 for females. (b) School menus contain 1/2 or more of protein needs in a single meal.
3. Adequate energy intake for growth/development and activity	(a) Adolescents on low caloric diets need to be advised that the protein needed for growth may be used for energy. (b) Plan for high carbohydrate intake so that protein is used for growth, not energy. (c) Determine energy to approach an accepted weight.
4. Achieve/maintain suggested weight	(a) Adjust energy intake after euglycemia is achieved. (b) Adjust insulin dosages. (c) Monitor weight regularly.
5. Watch for early symptoms of eating disorders	(a) Adolescents all have social pressures that may not be compatible with health aims, talk about these promptly.

TABLE 10. Nutrition Misconceptions in Athletics

Nutrition Misconceptions	Possible Effect on Athlete with IDDM
1. Protein foods are the most important for the athletic diet	Overemphasis on meat in the diet would also increase the fat in the diet. The recommended allowance of protein can easily be met by 3-5 oz of meat, 4 cups of low fat milk and 5-6 servings of grain products.
2. "Carbohydrate loading" enhances endurance in athletic events	The practice of eating high carbohydrate diets by athletes to increase glycogen stores is of no advantage to people with IDDM who normally eat high carbohydrate diets. Nor is it an advantage to athletes for short term events. The practice of fasting prior to the high carbodrate diet is hazardous to the person with IDDM and not recommended for other athletes.
3. Athletes need extra amounts of vitamins, minerals and amino acids, in general, multiple supplements	People with IDDM, who eat a variety of ordinary foods in amounts needed and take enough insulin, get no benefit from added supplements and risk possible harm.
4. Sports drinks "formulated to replace body fluids" are the best thirst quenchers, and increase performance capacity	Water is needed by athletes and every one and is the best thirst quencher and the best replacement for loss of body fluids. Added sugars in drinks may cause digestive disturbances that hinder athletic performance. Added minerals (electrolytes) in drinks may be of more harm than help when body water is lost.
5. Athletes need extra salt (sodium)	The practice of taking salt tablets is not recommended. Sodium is lost in sweat during exercise, especially when the environmental temperature is high, but eating more salty foods or more liberal salting of foods will replace losses. Any increase in salt intake must be accompanied by an increase of water. Note: Salt restriction and use of diuretics for weight loss is particularly dangerous.

cemia requires adjustment of food (increased) and long term insulin decrease.[5]

Prior to exercise an individual with IDDM may increase food intake or reduce insulin dosage to prevent hypoglycemic episodes. Because each individual reacts differently to changes in activity, blood glucose monitoring should be recommended.

For overweight individuals with NIDDM, exercise should be

viewed as an opportunity to expend energy and lose weight. Therefore, food consumption prior to exercise is not encouraged. If hypoglycemia results, insulin or oral medication should be reduced. Actual hypoglycemia probably will not occur if an individual is not taking insulin or oral medication, but patients often fear hypoglycemia and may experience a "false" hypoglycemic reaction.

Sporting events are of short duration (minutes) or involve sporadic intense activity (doubles tennis, football, baseball) but some involve intense prolonged activity (basketball, cycling, and long distance racing). Much of the energy of all events used is in training or practice and careful analysis of the intensity and duration is very important for the person with diabetes. An activity record (See Appendix II) can be used or even a video tape of the person can help estimate energy needs.

Easton adapted the Harker/Easton Method (Table 1) for the dog team drivers of the Alaskan Iditarod.[6] The intensity factor (Table 11) (called Iditarod Factor) was calculated to estimate additional needs based on the amount of clothing and gear carried and the long hours of racing. Some similar calculations are needed for long duration energy use of other sporting events or intense practice periods.

Dietary Treatment of Hypoglycemia

With the advent of tighter glucose control, episodes of hypoglycemia appear to be increased.[7] Although the tendency is often to over-treat or "over-prevent," swift treatment of hypoglycemia is necessary.

There is a great variance in detection of symptoms and the time necessary for the food eaten to correct hypoglycemia. The amount of fat, fiber, proteins and higher levels of saccharides (disaccharides and polysaccharides) all effect the length of time for glucose to become available without digestion. The use of glucose equivalents is now recommended.[8,9] Since sucrose (table sugar) has no glucose available before digestion, it is not the food of choice unless it is the only source of sugar available. If no glucose is readily available, the use of any sugar or sweetened soft drink is still advised if obtaining anything else would take more than fifteen minutes. The addition of sugar to orange juice is not recommended

TABLE 11. Harker/Easton Method of Estimating Energy Use Adapted for the Iditarod (6)

For energy use on an ordinary active day:

A. Usual energy needs: Multiply actual body weight in pounds by appropriate factor below:

Age	Fat	Normal Weight	Lean
Males	(20% BF*)	(15% BF)	(5% BF)
15-20	18	21	24
19-22	16	19	22
23-50	14	17	20
51-70	12	15	17
70+	10	12	14
Females	(25% BF)	(20% BF)	(10% BF)
15-18	15	18	21
19-22	13	16	19
23-50	12	15	18
51-70	10	12	14
70+	9	11	13

* Body Fat

B. Added energy use for Race Day: Iditarod Factor (IF) of 0.75 is calculated to compensate for additional energy needed per hour of the Race. This factor is applied to the weight of the person plus the weight of clothing (c) worn and gear (g) carried (c+g wt).

Calculation for Race Day

Body weight (lbs) X kcal per lb,(A) = Normal energy (kcal) use (based on age and degree of body fat) added to
[Body weight (lbs) + (c + g wt)] X 0.75 (I factor) X time (in hours) = Exertion energy use. (B)

Normal (active) energy use = _____kcal (A)

Exertion energy use   = _____kcal (B)

Total Race Day energy = _____kcal (A) + (B)

because the added sugar increases the electrolyte load in the gastro-intestinal tract and will not make glucose available any sooner.

The use of pure glucose is the treatment of choice but even predigested D-glucose may take 20 minutes for minimal response and 40 minutes to reach the maximum level.[8]

The use of milk is still encouraged for children as a snack to prevent hypoglycemic episodes and may still be a reasonable follow-up treatment after glucose tablets or fruit juice. All treatments do have caloric value and this must be considered to keep food intake, insulin, and weight control in balance.

The amount of glucose needed varies with the blood glucose level and the patient's size. The use of self-monitoring blood glucose before additional food or retreatment is necessary and the allowance of sufficient time for initial treatment to occur is essential.

Some amounts of foods necessary to produce approximately 15 grams of glucose before digestion are given in Table 12.

Usually an additional 10-15 grams of carbohydrate per half hour of exercise is adequate to prevent hypoglycemia during a moderate exercise program. However, a person who is in poor control and/or spilling ketones should not exercise until diabetes is in good control. Exercise can be used to lower blood glucose, especially following a meal.

Snacking prior to exercise often gives the patient the opportunity to overeat. Increased intake with exercise deletes the benefits of the program and decreases the long-term effects of training. Precise guidelines as to exercise timing and food intake should be given and physician monitoring is essential.

TABLE 12. Amounts of Foods Yielding Approximately 15 Grams of Glucose Before Digestion

Food	Amount for 14-16 gm glucose	Grams of fructose for same amount of food	kcal
Gelatin, flavored mix sweetened, prepared	1/4 c	*	210
Honey	2 Tb	18	130
Molasses, regular	7 Tb	18	350
Corn Syrup, light	3 1/2 Tb	3	210
Corn Syrup, high fructose	2 Tb	15	125
Apple juice	2 1/2 c	35	300
Orange juice (frozen, re-constituted)	1 1/4 c	14	138
Raisins	1/3 c	16	140
Soft Drink, Cola type	1 1/2 c	16	145
Gingerale	2 c	20	152
Thirst quenchers ("Gatorade")	2 1/2 c	13	150
Banana (2-1/2/lb)	3	9	300

* Sugar is present but data are lacking on amount

Source: Matthews, R.H., Pehrsson, P.R., Farhat-Sabet, M.: Sugar Content of Selected Foods: Individual and total sugars. USDA, Human Nutrition Information Services, Home Economics Research Report No. 48, 1987.

SECTION II: CHAPTER V
PREGNANCY AND LACTATION

General Description

The ideal situation for medical personnel who are supervising a woman with diabetes is that she presents herself before conception and is in good control before conception occurs. Good control of diabetes is complicated by pregnancy and requires constant medical supervision during the whole pregnancy and afterwards for the health of both the infant and mother.[10,11]

Dietary treatment is similar for women with IDDM whether or not they are pregnant,[12] but monitoring is especially important during pregnancy. Attention needs to be paid to nausea and food beliefs and so called cravings. During the first half of pregnancy, insulin requirement may drop 20-30%, and rise to 100% above pre-pregnancy during the second half.[13,14]

Three meals and three snacks are probably necessary and involve daily structured and carefully calculated and instructed diet plans such as the Exchange System or the Food Choice Plan.

In NIDDM, weight loss is usually a goal in treatment; however, this is not true in the individual who is pregnant or contemplating pregnancy. Rather, a maintenance weight should be attained prior to conception and a normal weight gain during pregnancy should be encouraged. The NIDDM patient if previously controlled with diet and oral agents may now require insulin to achieve and maintain near normal blood glucose levels.

Needs for Specific Nutrients During Pregnancy

Energy

Estimated energy needs have been based upon kcal/kgm body weight or simply described as so many additional kcals per day. Most authorities now consider that there is no difference in energy needs throughout the pregnancy and that the 80,000 kcal energy cost of the pregnancy can be met by a daily increase of 300 kcal over the amount needed by a non-pregnant woman.[3] If the pregnant woman decreases her activity from the level maintained before pregnancy, then her energy intake will need to be adjusted to prevent either too rapid or too much weight gain. Close monitoring of body weight is essential especially when the common 300 kcal/day increase is used.

During pregnancy an individual is more prone to hypoglycemia, especially during sleep. A bedtime feeding of complex carbohydrate and protein is encouraged to prevent hypoglycemia.

During the first trimester it is especially important to be alerted to and avoid the impending problem of starvation ketosis. This may result from a decrease in appetite, anorexia and/or vomiting. Hypoglycemia can occur frequently and without warning. Distribution of meals/snacks is important. The patient should have a through understanding of the diet and its rationale. The use of glucose monitoring with careful education and monitoring is generally recommended.

Current recommendations for total weight gain are 20-28 lbs. As previously indicated an estimated 300 kcal/day provides for energy needs to support this average weight gain. For the patient who is above recommended weight range, weight loss/maintenance at this time is not recommended and a weight gain of at least 20 lbs. is still usually advised. This weight gain should be evenly distributed through the prenatal period.

Protein

To meet increased protein needs a minimum of 10 grams per day above non-pregnant requirements are recommended for the entire pregnancy.[3] This additional protein is generally supplied without problem with the increase in foods for energy. The possibility of renal failure as a complicating factor in diabetes mellitus should not be ignored and protein intake should not be overly generous, should be of high quality, and sufficient energy must be available so that the protein is used for growth of fetus and maintenance of the mother rather than for energy.

The FAO/WHO recommendation for protein during pregnancy is less than that of the RDA's. Only 6 gm of protein/day increase is suggested by FAO/WHO.[12]

Vitamins and Minerals

In general the vitamin and mineral recommendations for the U.S. are higher than other countries. Whether this is a benefit or not is often debated.[12]

A calcium intake of 1,200 mg and 10 micrograms of Vitamin D are recommended daily. These recommendations are the same for pregnant women whether or not they have diabetes. With a variety of foods and 4 cups milk/day, these needs will be met. At times when milk or milk products are not tolerated, a calcium supplement is required.

The recommended dietary allowance (RDA) for iron for non-pregnant women is 15 mg/day.[3] An additional allowance of 15 mg of iron per day is recommended during pregnancy. This amount of iron cannot be met by diet, and a daily supplement probably is needed. The form of iron in food and the presence of other dietary components affect absorption and utilization of iron. High fiber diets or added fiber concentrates may inhibit or decrease the absorption of some minerals including iron.

The RDA for folic acid during pregnancy is 400 micrograms/day.[9] Folic acid is important and needs to be increased during pregnancy. If fresh vegetables and other foods are well chosen, sufficient amounts may be furnished without supplements.

A routine sodium restriction which was once commonly given to all pregnant women is no longer recommended. With the increase in blood and fluid volume, sodium needs are actually increased. However, a sodium restriction may be necessary when blood pressure is elevated or a great deal of swelling is noted. Moderation is the key and while a moderate to severe restriction is not indicated, the pregnant woman should not overdo her salt intake. A "no added salt" (3-5 gm) pattern may be desirable. This includes the avoidance of salt added to foods and foods high in sodium such as potato chips, cured meats, and fast foods.

The use of sweeteners for all people with diabetes is under a great deal of study.[13] Some experts recommend fructose and caution against the use of sucrose. At the present time pregnant women are advised to avoid saccharin use including saccharin sweetened soft drinks.

Constipation is often a problem during pregnancy especially for those taking an iron supplement. Regular exercise, adequate fluids and a variety of fresh fruits/vegetables and whole grains which add fiber to the diet assist in relieving constipation. However, too much fiber can affect the absorption of minerals and may even cause a colonic impaction.

During lactation, nutrient needs are only slightly higher than pregnancy. Primarily an increase in fluids and kilocalories are needed for milk production (1500-2000cc fluid per day and 500 kcal above non-pregnant intake) An additional 10 grams protein/day above non-pregnant levels is recommended. Recommendations for calcium are 1200 mg per day,[3] which can be provided by 4 cups of milk.

SECTION II: CHAPTER VI
GESTATIONAL DIABETES

Gestational diabetes mellitus (GDM) occurs in 2-3% of pregnancies. Dietary management is foremost in the treatment regimen with the primary goal being the achievement of euglycemia.[14]

The nutritional recommendations for the woman with GDM are the same as given for pregnancy for the woman with IDDM. Although the use of diet alone is often the treatment for GDM, some studies are showing possible advantages in the use of insulin. High fiber intakes should be encouraged, especially soluble fiber to aid in improving plasma glucose levels. Women utilizing glucose monitoring may be better able to monitor those foods having either a high or low glycemic response. Such monitoring may lead to improved postprandial blood glucose control.

Saccharin is not recommended for use.[13] The use of aspartame is still under debate. Some researchers are concerned that blood phenylalanine levels may be dangerously increased with aspartame.

Devising the meal plan for the GDM patient is no different than for the pregnant woman with IDDM. Three meals with a bedtime snack and/or 2 to 3 other snacks during the day should be included. To avoid large blood glucose excursions, food should be distributed evenly throughout the day. Controlling blood sugar may be difficult with the recommended increase in milk consumption for calcium because the minimum number of cups per day may provide an excess of simple sugars.

Successful pregnancy/delivery rests upon the achievement of a balance in diet, medication, and exercise which promotes the achievement of euglycemia while gaining the appropriate amount of weight. Utmost in the regimen is education of the patient, individualized meal planning, blood glucose monitoring as well as follow-up and support.

SECTION II: CHAPTER VII
IMPAIRED GLUCOSE TOLERANCE
AND MATURITY ONSET DIABETES IN YOUTH

Impaired Glucose Tolerance (IGT)

The dietary management of people with impaired glucose tolerance is the diet appropriate to the age level and condition of the patient. This may involve weight loss, gain, or weight maintenance. The dietary strategies for IGT are no different from those of the person with NIDDM. These can be found in the appropriate sections of this reference.

Maturity Onset Diabetes in Youth (MODY)

Maturity Onset Diabetes in Youth is an unusual condition which requires different nutritional strategies than those used for youth with IDDM. Treatment for IDDM is a source of exogenous insulin. In MODY, weight correction is indicated and hypoglycemia is not a constant threat. Some weight correction and control strategies are indicated in Section V. The individual will experience similar social pressures of youth and social support is indicated. Caloric contribution of foods in terms of peer acceptable foods is of major importance and energy intake can sometimes be controlled by serving size alone. Desired foods in appropriate amounts may be used to replace needed foods in order to accomplish weight loss.

REFERENCES

1. Taras, H.L., Nadar P.R., Sallis, J.F., Patterson, T.L. and Rupp, J.W.: Early childhood diet: Recommendations of pediatric health care providers. J Am Diet Assoc 88:1417, Nov 1988.

2. Pipes, P.L.: Nutrition in Infancy and Childhood. St. Louis: Times Mirror Mosby College Publishing, 1985.

3. Food and Nutrition Board, National Research Council. Recommended Dietary Allowances, 10th revised ed.: Washington, D.C., National Academy of Sciences, 1989.

4. Anderson, B.J., Wold, F.M., Burkhart, M.H., Cornell, R.G., Bacon, G.E.: Effects of peer-group intervention on metabolic control of adolescents with IDDM. Diabetes Care 12:3:179, Mar 1989.

5. Allen, D.B., MacDonald, M.J.: Preventing postexercise late-onset hypoglycemia. Practical Diabetology 8:1, Jan/Feb 1989.

6. Easton, P.S.: Food considerations for Iditarod drivers. In Turner, A.A., ed.: The Iditarod Artic Sports Medicine/Human Performance Guide, 2nd ed. Anchorage: 1989.

7. Simonson, D.C., Tamborlane, W.V., DeFronzo, R.A., and Sherwin, R.S.: Intensive insulin therapy reduces counterregulatory hormone responses to hypoglycemia in patients with Type I diabetes. Ann Intern Med 103:185:Aug 1985.

8. Wheeler, M.L. Comment: Treatment of insulin reactions in diabetes. Diabetes Spectrum 1:5:307, Nov/Dec 1988.

9. Brodows, R.G., Williams C., and Amatruda, J.M.: Treatment of insulin reactions in diabetes. JAMA 252:3378, 1984.

10. Langer, O.: Scientific rationale of management of diabetes in pregnancy. Diabetes Care 11:1:69, Nov/Dec 1988.

11. Burns, E.M.: Diabetes mellitus and pregnancy. Nursing Clinics of North America 18:4:673, Dec 1983.

12. Whitehead, R.G.: Pregnancy and Lactation, Chapter 49 in Modern Nutrition in Health and Disease, 7th ed. Edited by Shils, M.E. and Young, V.R. Philadelphia, Lea and Febiger, 1988.

13. Anderson, J.W.: Nutrition management of diabetes mellitus. Chapt 57 in Modern Nutrition in Health and Disease, 7th ed. Edited by Shils, M.E. and Young, V.R., Philadelphia, Lea and Febiger, 1988.

14. Drexel, H., Bichler, A., Salier, S., Breier, C., Lisch, H.J., Braunsteiner, H., Patsch, J.R.: Prevention of perinatal prenatal morbidity by tight metabolic control in gestational diabetes mellitus. Diabetes Care 11:10:761, Nov/Dec 1988.

Section III:
Nutrition in the Adult and Aging Years

INTRODUCTION

Adults with diabetes cannot be considered to belong to one group of people or even to two groups according to the type of diabetes, IDDM or NIDDM. There need to be several subcategories according to state of control, evidence of complications and duration of the disease. Some of these categories are listed in Tables 13 and 14 with suggestions for dietary counseling. Other tables consider the emotional climate and feelings of some people and some caregivers.

Further information covering dietary prescriptions for adults, both at home and in the hospital are given in Section I, Chapter III.

SECTION III: CHAPTER I
ADULT YEARS

General Considerations of Adults

The adult with diabetes has been given many messages from society. Most of these are negative and frightening. Table 15 lists some of these for the adult with IDDM and Table 16 for the adult with NIDDM. Dietary management for the adult is difficult because of his/her many roles. The usual request for dietary advice is for something that "fits my lifestyle," however some patients may deny the ability to make any dietary adjustment at all.

Some adults have much misinformation about the cause and management of diabetes. Many "sugar myths" are believed by adults with diabetes or by their friends and families. They may believe that eating excess sugar causes diabetes, that sugar is a poison, and/or that only "natural" sugars should be eaten. A great deal of confu-

TABLE 13. Implications for Dietary Counseling for Individuals with IDDM

Group/Category	Approaches
1. IDDM, newly diagnosed	Determine appropriate diet prescription with frequent nutrition counseling and follow-up. Adjust diet to prevent weight gain as control improves. Limit restrictions to only the essential ones.
2. IDDM, long standing	
A. Out of control	(a) Recalculate prescription, ascertain food intake.
B. Complications	(b) Adjust food spacing or actual nutrients according to complication. Instruct caretakers to monitor nutrient intake.
C. Other diseases concurrent with DM	(c) See Section IV for diets for specific disorders. Make only necessary restrictions.
D. Life style changes	(d) Recalculate prescription. Determine and monitor intake. Make practical suggestions - recommend social agencies, convenience foods.
3. IDDM, long standing reasonably good control	Reinforce behavior, ascertain intake to make prescription or chart agree with actual intake. Protect against "scare" advice and old cumulative prohibitions.
4. IDDM gaining weight	Recalculate prescription, ascertain adherence and problems. Explain how to lower insulin/lower food intake. Ascertain if hypoglycemia is "over-treated" or over-aggressively prevented.

sion occurs in information about the types of diabetes and the hypoglycemic agents prescribed. Equally great confusion occurs about the role of diet in the prevention of diseases such as atherosclerosis and cancer.

The professional treating the adult needs to determine which food beliefs patients hold and their feelings about food. The reported food intake may be very different from usual food intake. One author noticed that food intake recalls reflect what the patients know rather than what they actually eat because she got identical recalls year after year.

Health professionals striving to give their patients the best possi-

TABLE 14. Implications for Dietary Counseling for People with NIDDM

Group/Category	Implications
1. NIDDM, newly diagnosed	
A. Stable high weight or gaining	(a) Candidate for strict dietary management. Careful calculation and recalculation of prescription.
B. Losing weight	(b) Needs constant reinforcement. Realistic goals for weight loss. Variety of food plans may be helpful.
C. Not overweight	(c) Strict monitoring of food intake and exercise. Food spacing important.
2. NIDDM, long term under control with diet alone	Reinforce behavior. Adjust for life style changes. Don't impose unnecessary restrictions.
3. NIDDM, long term under control with oral agents (not obese)	May be a candidate for another trial of diet alone. Good nutrition history and monitoring.
4. NIDDM long term under control with oral agents or insulin (obese)	Watch aggressive prevention of hypoglycemia. May be candidate for very strict M.D./R.D. supervised diet.

ble advice may give so many restrictions and conditions that the resulting dietary pattern is impossible to follow. Priority ranking of different aspects of dietary advice is imperative. Table 17 shows some dietary recommendations and approaches for adults.

What is necessary? Possible? In what order? Changes in food intake are constantly occurring. People will experiment with new foods, different restaurants, and eating at different times. All people must constantly decide what to eat, when to eat, and what not to eat.

Food is important in religion, hospitality, diplomacy, business and families. Food cues are connected with all of these. Additional food cues abound in advertising of all kinds and in the 24 hour accessibility of food at home, in restaurants, or even vending machines. One can drive to a store or restaurant at any time or even order a variety of foods delivered at all hours of the day or night. Few people have no refrigerator or freezer. Controlling these cue induced cravings or appetites is difficult for everyone and particularly difficult for those with diabetes who are on restrictive diets.

TABLE 15. Social Messages for IDDM Patients Affecting Food Choices

Impact	Messages	Solution
Often parents (and the child as well) blame themselves for transmitting the disease. The individual may blame himself for the disease progression since it is a nutrition related disease.	Guilt	Health professionals need to explain pathology and physiology and causes of disease as well as treatment regimen and balancing of diet - activity - insulin.
Hosts often find people with special food needs a "nuisance" and they may not be invited or resented. This adds stress to patient in meeting treatment regimens. (Patients may encourage this as an attention getting device.) Some people still think of diabetes as contagious!!!	Unwelcome at social occasions	Teach management of food intake; allow substitutions and/or adjust insulin dose. Have written material explaining patient's ability to choose ordinary foods in appropriate amounts. This could be addressed to family members or friends.
Many friends and employers think that hypoglycemic reactions make a person undependable or dangerous.	Undependable socially and at work.	Have patient learn self glucose monitoring and demonstrate ability to prevent crises. Written material is also useful here as is record of episodes of high or low blood glucose.
The complications of diabetes produce undue fear often from ignorance. If they occur, patient may be "written off" as responsible for the condition.	Fear of future ill health	Patient support groups need to know danger and treatment. Denial is probably most dangerous attitude.
The hereditary factors are not known sufficiently by the general public. Improper dietary practices are often blamed or parent may be told it's from "his" or "her" family.	Health of children	Education of genetic risk and predisposition - Differentiation between nutrition treatment and causes of disease.

Often, the patient is unjustly criticized by family and medical personnel for "cheating."

There is no perfect diet. Some people like the challenge and rigidity of the Exchange System, some like the flexibility of other plans (see Section I, Chapter III). All diets need careful planning

TABLE 16. Social Messages for NIDDM Patients Affecting Food Choices

Impact	Messages	Solution
Patient is blamed for cause of disease especially when associated with obesity of patient or may place guilt on caregiver or family member.	Guilt	Teaching, understanding of society's present obesssion with thinness and positive and negative effects this has on the weight conscious. Teach serving sizes and food substitutes.
Disease may be considered to be moral or physical weakness of the patient. May be pampered, feared or ignored by friends and/or family. Food may be used as a weapon.	Weakness	Patients need strategies to resist urging of family and friends to consume greater amounts of "good foods" or specialty items.
The sociability of food may be denied. Hosts consider small serving or food refusal as insulting. Host may "know" what patient should eat.	Hospitality denied	Help patient to state openly and often what and how much can be eaten. Teach them to entertain and still maintain dietary management. Teach serving sizes and food substitutions.
Type of diabetes may contribute to patient's own denial and reluctance to manage food intake. Taking extra oral hypoglycemic agents to combat dietary indiscretions may result.	Has a mild form of disease	Recognition of this attitude and management strategies are needed. Home glucose monitoring may be needed.
Patient's wish for large amounts of food and frequent meals may be judged "ridiculous" by normal weight people.	Can't be hungry so soon after a meal	Food cues, hyperinsulinemia and hunger should all be explained. Dilution of food with water or cellulose may be useful.

and constant readjusting similar to the fitting of clothes. This does not mean that the authors think there is any "one size fits all diet" or that there is any real substitution for constant dietary advice or monitoring.

Nutritional supplements are not usually needed for obese persons with diabetes.[1] A low dose multivitamin with iron may be comforting to physicians and patients alike. A history of supplemental nutrient intakes should be taken to ensure that overdoses do not occur. Iron supplements can cause constipation. Reasons for low levels of iron in the blood should be explored before iron supplements are used.

TABLE 17. Dietary Recommendations for Adults

Recommendation(s)	Approach(es)
1. Obtain glycemic control as near normal as possible.	(a) Dietary management (b) NIDDM - weight loss as little as 10-20 lbs. Hypoglycemic agents may be necessary for some NIDDM patients.
2. Prevent and/or minimize complications (i.e. neuropathies, retinopathy)	Dietary management as well as changes in prescriptions and strategies are needed with frequent monitoring.
3. Obtain/maintain adequate nutritional intake	There is no real standard of nutrient intake; however, good nutrition is met by most dietary regimens and should probably be a secondary goal.
4. Participate in regular exercise program	(a) Evaluate each patient individually and design appropriate regimen. Example - neuropathy may make walking a painful exercise and must be controlled. (b) Instruct patient on dietary intake, placement of meals, etc. for prevention of hypoglycemia.

Calculations of Energy Needs

Although estimation of energy needs for all people with diabetes is difficult and usually inaccurate, such calculations for the elderly person may be even further from the truth. The use of formulas especially those based on skin fold thickness and/or the adapted Harris Benedict formula, may be more time consuming than necessary (see Section I, Chapter III). The following conservative methods are suggested:

1. Obtain height and weight history. Evidence of edema needs to be noted. Weight should be accurately measured at least monthly at onset of disease for evidence of deterioration of control.
2. Estimates of usual food intake with use of observation and histories, changes in food preparation such as decreased use of sugar and/or fats, or smaller servings should be noted and ef-

fect estimated. Skipped, refused or regurgitated meals need to be calculated.

3. Changes in energy use such as sitting or walking, fever, and stress need to be noted.
4. Changes in liquid consumption (often not considered foods) should be noted. Beverages with sweeteners or creamers should be estimated.

The above data can help the practitioner more accurately determine nutrient use, especially if the patient is new or rarely observed. There is no real substitute for careful, frequent, critical observation of the patient. The absence of accurate height and weight and food consumption data should not be tolerated in even minimal health care.

The dangerous assumption that the energy prescription is correct and the patient "wrong" must be considered. It is true that some people do not follow orders even if they understand them; it is also true that many estimates, particularly of energy needs and use, are wrong. It is not unusual for all patients to be given so called 1000 kcal Diabetic Diets regardless of whether this is a fasting level for the active 6'2" man or weight gain inducing level for the 4'0" sedentary woman.

The changes in the Exchange Lists (See Table 3) have made many old prescriptions that used them obsolete. However, the food intake may not need to be changed, just recalculated and explained (see Section I, Chapter V). Continuing dietary counseling is necessary and probably cost effective.[2]

SECTION III: CHAPTER II
AGING YEARS

The definition of "elderly" is difficult. Many physical changes occur with aging and these vary greatly with individuals. To clinically declare a person of 60, 65 or 70 elderly denies these differences. For the purpose of description, this section will be divided into the young elderly, usually under 70, and the elderly. The young elderly described here are able to care for themselves physically and are usually financially secure but may have limited ability to withstand inflation. They tend to be alert and interested. They often are valuable community leaders in diabetes groups, hospital auxiliaries, and politics. To date, the number of women has far exceeded men but the number of men is growing.

The young elderly with IDDM of long standing may have some complication or condition which will require new or revised treatment. Changes in the treatment of diabetes, use of self glucose monitoring, and more accurate determination of actual food intake can be learned and often benefit the person. If the adjustment and control has been good, radical changes are not advised. The conditions in Table 18 must be considered.

These young elderly usually read and hear medical advice and may compulsively try to prevent all possible conditions. They deserve inexpensive sources of accurate diet information. For example, the "alar scare" concerning apples need not be a high priority with them. Qualified evaluation of public information on diabetes must be available for the concerned well-read patient.

Home Care of the Elderly

The diet of young elderly living alone has to be carefully tailored to lifestyle and availability of food. Realistic recreational use of food and alcoholic beverages should be considered. The presence or onset of complications such as retinopathy may make the measuring of food and medications difficult. Such changes are often so gradual that the patient does not realize they occur. Even the serving size of a food may appear smaller as the eyesight is impaired. The minimal competencies at least should be tested at each follow-up session (Section I). If patients wear reading glasses then they should always wear these glasses to measure and serve food.

Usually in NIDDM the patient should not be given oral agents or insulin until after multiple, well-monitored strategies are tried unless symptoms require their use. Support groups and reinforcement visits are helpful. The need to start over, try something new, find a new pattern is probably what leads to much of the faddist appeal. These needs can be met in a safer manner with good medical care including food preparation techniques and social skills. (See Alternative Strategies in Section I.) Tables 13 and 14 provide some implications for counseling people with diabetes mellitus.

The person with IDDM usually has constant need of tight control. The changes listed above affect these patients as well. The person with IDDM if well taught can make temporary adjustments but regularity of schedule and weight control is important.

On the positive side, patients with diabetes of longstanding and

TABLE 18. Possible Effects of and Remedies for Conditions in Diabetes Mellitus in the Elderly

Conditions Common in Elderly	Effects on Diabetes Mellitus	Remedy
1. Change in energy use	Decreased metabolic rate	Help patient understand that expected weight loss may be less than desired.
2. Activity decreased as result of aging	Causes weight gain	See weight control strategies.
3. Other medical conditions	May have difficulty eating, handling food	Food plan modified, cooking lessons. Prioritize advice according to the most critical condition.
4. Retirement A. Different kinds of stress B. Different amounts of activity C. Decrease in medical attention	(a) Changes in schedules and support systems (b) Old diet prescription inappropriate (c) May have antiquated beliefs and advice	(a) Review food schedules - try different plans. (b) Recalculate diet prescription. (c) Take and record detailed diet history.
5. Many medications often self-prescribed such as laxatives and vitamins	May have food and drug interactions, use of medications with sugar or alcohol.	Instruction both written and oral to patient and caregivers about kinds and doses of medicine.
6. Fall prey to faddists, quacks, expensive "miracle" cures	Expensive, may forego necessary treatment, visits for diet monitoring, may actually take toxic doses of vitamins.	Instruction both written and oral to patient and caregivers about kinds and doses of medicine.
7. Alcohol intake	May affect total intake and cause weight gain.	Need to be monitored and not denied unless absolutely necessary as in addiction.

TABLE 18 (continued)

Conditions Common in Elderly	Effects on Diabetes Mellitus	Remedy
8. Lack of understanding, multiple advice	May overdo "good" advice such as fiber intake.	Written repeated advice about keeping good food intake records.
9. Socialization restricted. Food restricted. Loss of spouse, family, friends	Increased use of sugars, convenience foods.	Review restaurant choices and serving sizes.
10. Decreased incentive	May find purchase of and storage of fresh food difficult.	Monitor food records and adjust plans for this.

in good control can be delightful and helpful when some of the guilt for not following antiquated advice is removed. The young elderly have adapted to a larger number of changes and are often willing, able, and eager to make positive changes in their lives.

Some sample menus are found in the Appendixes. Note that these are restricted in energy (kcal) but allow some foods traditionally forbidden. Fruit juice is omitted because of the frequency of "overdose." Whole fruit is allowed and may give added benefits because of the soluble fibers. Fruit and fruit juice both are limited at breakfast because of the common morning glucose elevations. Of course, if the person wants juice it should be included and serving sizes taught.

IDDM Hospitalized Patient

The practice of hospitalizing patients with diabetes to adjust insulin and diet makes sense in terms of the necessity for tight control and availability of medical personnel for monitoring and education. However, the differences in hospital routines, amount of rest, stresses, different food patterns, and different exercise patterns mean that additional education in terms of post hospitalization changes is absolutely necessary. Patients need to know that a diet prescription needs checking and adjustments as do other prescriptions (see Section I, Chapter III).

The increase in certified diabetes education programs has increased amounts of third party payments for diet education. An increasing number of dietitians are joining the Diabetes Education

Practice Groups of the American Dietetic Association and/or becoming certified Diabetic Educators and becoming professional members of the American Diabetes Association.

Hospitalizations for other conditions, such as fevers, surgery, and injuries, all require changes in dietary treatment. Rarely should restricted diets for weight loss be used during these periods although weight gain should be avoided as well. The dietary prescription on record or quoted by the patient is usually not what the patient has been eating. At admission, a diet history, and/or 24-hour recall may be useful. (See Appendix III and Section I, Chapter III.) This is best taken by a dietitian who knows the correct probing questions and therefore achieves a less "guilt driven recall." Equally or more useful may be careful food and glucose monitoring and determination of insulin needs. Monitoring of actual intake and recalculation of energy needs is necessary.

Patients, significant others, and floor personnel can learn to monitor accurately intake of food as they do fluid balance if proper forms and instructions are given. Translation of intake records to nutrients is often best done by dietitians although some computer programs do exist (see Nutrient Analysis, Section VI). "Calorie count" is the term used by most hospitals to indicate food consumption records. These are a necessity for all patients with diabetes. The old practice of replacing foods not eaten or vomited is probably still appropriate as is the old formula of replacement food for the hospitalized patient of 100% carbohydrate, 50% protein, and 10% fat.

A menu pattern for liquid diets is included in Section IV, under "Special Diets." The advantages of using commercial formulas are:

1. Sanitation can be controlled.
2. Measurements of intake are easier.
3. Reluctance to use sugar and radically forbidden foods is overcome.

The disadvantages are:

1. Expense is greater.
2. Unrealistic nutritional qualities given to formula preparations compared to formulas prepared from foods.

3. Flavor and consistency may be unacceptable.
4. Unrealistic evaluation of nutrient contribution and adequacy; therefore patient kept on regimen too long.
5. Patients may be initially upset with change in nutrient composition or food texture.

The Older Elderly

The older elderly usually have less physical and social flexibility. Changes, if necessary, in the diet often must be explained to caretakers, relatives or friends. Changes in serving sizes are an effective way of modifying intake without disrupting lifestyle.

The attention to and possible consequences of diabetes has often been a source of power to the elderly. They may have been given or demanded dietetic foods, special meal times, and patterns. If these are not counterproductive to treatment then these patterns may best be left alone. Reinforcing such myths should be watched. Multiple dietary restrictions are difficult and the major needs should be identified and treated in priority order. (See Section IV.) Multiple restrictions may result in actual malnutrition.

The occurrence of debilitating conditions are even more likely to happen in this age group. Decreased mobility and eyesight affect food procurement, preparation and serving sizes.

Most home health agencies employ dietitians at least part-time. Other medical personnel give dietary advice as well. All of this advice coupled with years of belief, advice, and learning may be conflicting and confusing to everyone concerned. Explicit written food intake plans should be developed with the patient, explained to caretakers and neighbors if necessary. Monitoring of effect and adherence to these plans must occur to prevent starvation, overeating, or lack of socialization. Cost of food and religious foods are of major importance. Food preparation, storage, and ability to procure food are all of major importance. Physical and financial complications abound.

Lowered levels of immunity, resistance to infection and possibly even reduced nutrient utilization can occur. Vitamins, minerals, and/or protein supplements should be a last resort, not first ordered.

The authors suggest that at least 4 hours by competent dietitians in several well spaced sessions are necessary for individual diet instruction of all elderly patients. Group instruction is often confusing for them. Support groups can aid or further confuse, depending on the leadership of the group. The elderly are far more adaptable than caregivers often think.

NIDDM Hospitalized Patient

NIDDM patients who are not taking insulin and not debilitated usually should not have between-meal and bedtime feedings and should learn the spacing of meals in order to allow blood glucose to return to normal (3 to 4 hours between meals).

The patient who has had diabetes for several years and who is hospitalized for some other reason needs help in adjusting to fever, surgery, etc., but should also, if able, play an active part in dietary choices. Standard dietary patterns may be very distressing. Equally distressing may be valid use of traditionally forbidden foods such as table sugar in liquid diets. The patient needs to understand the role of carbohydrates and the glucose contribution of various foods.

Multiple restrictions may actually require severe limitations of food intake. Often new instructions or restrictions are added to old beliefs and advice reducing intake to a dangerous level. For example, an elderly Jewish patient was given a low sodium, low fat prescription. When these were added to his previous prohibition of sugar and his religious beliefs, he literally starved.

The elderly patient newly diagnosed as NIDDM should be carefully monitored to see if restricted serving sizes alone may not accomplish necessary control. Absolute prohibition of treats, especially party or recreational foods, may be very distressing and unnecessary. Small plates and small servings may suffice.

This last very conservative approach has received criticism from some health care providers because they say it will not be approved by health care inspectors. Efforts should be made to change the regulations rather than deny the patient an improved quality of life.

The elderly person with NIDDM presents a problem in terms of lack of activity, and weight control. Total energy contribution of food regardless of other considerations may be the only or best way of management. Again, the belief of the caregiver, patient, and family must be considered and education given. Restriction of sugar and exercise with the often prescribed increase in fiber may actually cause constipation and great discomfort. Sugars ferment in the gastrointestinal tract system and may have a laxative effect.

The use of insulin and/or oral agents for the patient with NIDDM:

1. Will increase energy available if improved glycemic control occurs and therefore make patients gain weight on the same amounts of food.
2. May increase patient's hunger and make low energy diets more difficult to follow.
3. Can effect a rapid lowering of blood glucose to give the patient discomfort and feelings of hypoglycemia even though physiological hypoglycemia is not present.
4. May encourage over-aggressive prevention of hypoglycemia.

If weight gain is not occurring and the patient's condition is not affecting care (bed sores, moving, heat rashes, etc.), the elderly patient with diabetes can usually be managed more happily, economically, and efficiently with small serving sizes of regular foods, limited between meal snacks, artificially sweetened beverages and as few oral agents or as little insulin as possible.

Dietary management of the older person with diabetes in long-term care facilities requires:

1. Development or adjustment of prescription. (Note: Basal energy expenditure calculations and skinfold measurement are not advised). Weight monitoring, accurate weight/height determination, observation and frequent accurate weights are essential.
2. Reasonable adaptation of food type for prevention of complications through dietary means. Decreases in saturated fat may be of little consequence. It may be useful to calculate fats and sugar for limited use rather than forbid them.
3. Regular portion controlled meals and replacement of food not eaten or regurgitated is appropriate.

SECTION III: CHAPTER III
REGIONAL, ETHNIC AND RELIGIOUS FOOD PATTERNS

Regional and ethnic food patterns require study by health professionals. It is necessary to realize that not all members of the group follow the same patterns. With the large number of convenience foods available as well as the great variety of restaurants of all types, some aspects of so-called ethnic and regional patterns are often adopted by people far removed from the group originating the pattern. Young children especially are exposed to a variety of foods in schools as well as in advertisements. Sometimes they deny liking the food of their parents.

Some religious groups have allowed and/or forbidden foods and these too need to be studied by dietary advisors. The Jewish food patterns given later in this chapter are an example of strict rules which may apply to some people, be traditional in some families or be used as patterns for celebrations and family gatherings.

Even though many religions allow the patient dispensation when ill, the health professional should make every effort to allow the patient to follow the desired pattern if that is the patient's wish.

Table 19 gives some ideas about ethnic food groups which may be helpful in giving advice to patients from these groups or people who eat in ethnic restaurants. The size of servings is very important. Some hostesses only feel gracious if a great deal of food is served and people who pay a large amount of money for food expect large amounts for their money.

Mixed dishes such as those made with rices and pastas, stews, and soups can hide as much fat as some meats contribute even though meats are given more attention today.

Kosher Foods

Jewish patients who adhere to dietary laws have problems with foods on a restricted sodium regimen. Kosher meat is treated with salt to remove the blood. (Although patients have a dispensation for medical reasons, use of non-koshered meat is often an unnecessary psychological hindrance.) The following suggestions were advanced by Vivian Witkoff, M.S., R.D. in 1976.

TABLE 19. Characteristics of Ethnic Foods Important to People with Diabetes Mellitus

Group Description	Foods to Recommend	Foods to Limit or Avoid
Cuban: Use large amounts of pork and other high fat meats. Use few raw vegetables and many legumes. Like very sweet desserts.	Chicken dishes (do not eat skin). White rice and black beans (often served together).	Avoid flan and other desserts made with condensed milk. Cut portions of Cuban sandwiches and limit amounts of dressing and sauces. Limit serving size of chicken/rice, fried pork and beef and luncheon meat such as ham.
Mexican: Use many vegetables and legumes and highly spiced foods.	Steamed corn tortillas, beans in soft tortilla, black bean soup, gespacho, chicken with vegetables.	Watch serving size of fritos, fried tortillas, refried beans, extra cheese, tortilla chips with guacamole and nachos.
Chinese: Many vegetables, fried foods. Meat and fat in fried rice. High in salt. There are several different kinds of Chinese food which vary in spices.	White or brown steamed rice. Mixed vegetables, steamed dumpling, chicken and egg dishes - not fried.	Avoid egg rolls and fried foods. Limit size of servings. Limit duck dishes (fat).
Italian: Large amounts of oil and cheese. Often high in salt and fat.	Bread sticks, pastas with vegetables, steamed mussels, broth soups, fruit ices, pastas with small amount of sauce.	Garlic buttered bread, limit parmesan and romano cheeses, sauces with meat balls. Limit antipasto with anchovies and olives. Limit amounts of salad dressing and sauce. Avoid fetticini Alfredo and limit lasagna, canoloni.
French: Usually foods are sauteed and served with sauces. So-called "French fried" foods are not traditional French foods.	"New cuisine" foods with lighter sauces and often smaller servings.	Limit serving size and amount of sauce. Avoid rich desserts or eat fruit, fruit ices or sherberts.

Group Description	Foods to Recommend	Foods to Limit or Avoid
Thai: Lighter than Chinese and may be spicy. Usually can choose spiciness. Control less wise choices by smaller servings	Broth based soups, fish, squid, shellfish, poultry, (except duck), lean beef, white rice, vegetables and noodles.	Avoid foods covered with batter and /or fried. Limit coconut oil and dishes with coconut milk. Limit fried rice.
Japanese: Use much fish and many vegetables. Food often cooked at table. Be careful of raw fish because of sanitation.	Broth soups (miso), chicken, white rice, stir fried vegetables if not too much fat. Choose chicken, shrimp, tofu, cooked fish.	Tempura using fat. Any deep fried or foods covered with batter and fried, as in appetizers.

1. The dietitian should write the Union of Orthodox Jewish Congregations of America in New York, for one of its free booklets, such as Kashruth, Handbook for Home and School. This booklet presents a brief review of the guidelines and basic Kashruth information.

2. Dietitians and physicians should consider the following suggestions for patients who follow strict dietary laws and are on sodium restricted regimens. Since preparation of "koshered" meat involves two steps, meat butchered under ritualistic conditions and the removal of blood usually with the use of salt:

   a. Reduce the amount of meat allowed and permit small amounts of "kosher" meat.

   b. When a health problem exists, it is permissible to broil "kosher slaughtered" meat instead of salting. If the patient desires a pot roast, the meat can be broiled until it is one-half cooked, rinsed and then stewed or roasted.

   c. Suggest a consultation with the butcher to see if wholesale cuts can be "koshered" (salt added in the butcher shop). If this is possible, the patient can buy an inside cut. This would satisfy the requirements of koshering the meat and the diet prescription since sodium is not absorbed to that depth. (Note: This would not apply to chicken in the State of Florida. All Kosher chicken is shipped in from out of state. To meet the specific requirements of "koshering," the chicken is "koshered" by salting at the plant.)

3. The dietitian and physician should encourage the patient, when there is a conflict between the principles of the diet and the religious regulations, to discuss the problem with his rabbi to consider effecting a practical compromise.

SECTION III: CHAPTER IV
TRAVEL

Dietary advice to the person with diabetes mellitus who travels, of course, depends on what kind of diabetes is involved, status of control, and reasons for and frequency of travel.

The person who travels frequently for business reasons needs to meet the adequacy level competencies in Section I. This person needs to know how to adjust for time changes and sleep patterns as well as for stress levels and scheduled delays. With today's emphasis on fitness and low caloric foods, appropriate foods are usually available but the pressures of business meals and banquets may be considerable.

All travel involves the need for planning and management and some suggestions are given below. Note: Detailed printed travel tips are available from the American Diabetes Association and several other sources and patients should be advised to secure these and check them with health care team.

Air Travel

Most major airlines have some sort of special menus for special conditions. This usually involves at least 24-hours notice and notifying the cabin personnel of the order when boarding. The meals for people with diabetes may be listed "Diabetic," "Low Calorie" and sometimes even "Low Carbohydrate." Kosher and vegetarian meals may also be available.

These special meals are often more tasty than the regular fare but they may vary from 250 kcal to nearly a thousand. The person may not choose to be publicly declared "Diabetic," the meal may not be aboard or the schedule or flight changed. In these cases the regular meal can often be eaten with few changes such as omitting the butter and/or dessert. The servings are smaller than usual servings. (See Tables 20 and 21.)

Flights without meals usually have some food and/or beverages available and a ''meal'' can be chosen from them. Sometimes two

TABLE 20. Comparison of Some Airline Meals*

Breakfast

Regular	Est kcal	Diabetic	Est kcal
Orange Juice 4 oz	63	Tator Tots (6)	100
Crumb Cake	164	Scrambled Eggs	95
Scrambled Eggs	95	Grilled Tomato (1/2)	25
Sausage Links (2)	265	Roll	92
Potato Patty	72	Butter	30
Butter	30	1/4 Melon	57
Total	689	Total	399

Snack

Cheese and Peanut Butter Crackers	205	Crackers, 2 pkg	160
Fig Newtons	53	Cheese, 2 Wedges	106
Apple (lg)	100	Apple (lg)	100
Total	358		366

Lunch

Lasagna	290	Baked Chicken	225
Green Salad	20	Carrots, Green Beans	35
Salad Dressing	52	Green Salad	20
Crackers	120	"Diet" Dressing	16
Butter	30	Banana (lg)	125
Cake	250		
Total	762	Total	421

* These are estimates for actual meals served passengers on a major airline.

TABLE 21. Snacks to Substitute for Airline Meal

Foods	kcal
Peanuts, Roasted 1 oz	170
Milk, White 8 oz	150
Apple or Orange Juice, 6 oz	94
Total	414

Note: Artificial "creams" or half and half
       equal 20 kcal/Tbsp (appr)

meals will be served within four hours so caution must be used in this way as well. The food eaten as a snack, because of delayed service, or as a substitute must still be considered as part of the prescribed intake.

Car Travel

Planning is easier when travelling by car, but fatigue from riding or driving may be conducive to more food being consumed than actually needed. Sleep, exercise, and elimination schedules may be interrupted. Again, planning is necessary and the ability to eat part of a serving or forego dessert (even if included in price) is necessary. Here, the constant food cues of advertising and the large servings of food in places serving travelers must be dealt with carefully. Carrying of food in a cooler is often wise and exercise stops may be necessary for maintaining energy use as well as comfort.

Ship or Cruise Travel

During the last few years, exercise opportunities have increased on cruise ships. Some lines offer "fitness" cruises and special menu advice. However, there is still a tendency for cruise patrons to overeat and overindulge in alcohol, and to spend most of their trip sitting.

The person with diabetes going on a cruise needs to be willing to forego food, meals or a course even if "it's paid for." One solution to allow for "treats" and a festive feeling is to really learn food equivalents and eat only the course or food actually desired. Walking "stairs" instead of using elevators, and scheduled exercise even if only walking on deck or between common areas is helpful. Weight maintenance for the person with NIDDM is probably possible; much weight loss is very difficult.

SECTION III: CHAPTER V
DIABETES INSTRUCTION IN OTHER COUNTRIES

Recent interviews with dietitians in Canada, England, the Netherlands, Denmark and Finland show that the instruction methods vary from dietitian to dietitian as they do in the United States. All have the same goals of helping the patient adapt to a normal lifestyle. The natural food patterns of all these countries appear to be slightly more uniform in terms of foods chosen and eating times. However, the growth in "American Style" food items, fast foods and snack items is tremendous and greatly influences the youth and young people. Food cues for these items and changes in stated meal times are necessary and complicate diet instruction. In general, the equivalent lists are less complicated than the ADA Exchange System, and all countries studied have the need for instruction materials for minority groups with patterns and languages different from the majority of population.

The dietitians in all of these countries who shared their expertise had innovative techniques such as large supplies of labels available and all commented on the need for repeated classes with follow up sessions.

The leaders in diabetic research have many opportunities for sharing research findings and often contribute to journals in countries other than where they live. Nutrition research is included but the study of actual food intake and dietary counseling is still too limited.

The Canadian Diabetic Association and other health agencies publish many pamphlets about nutrition. Instructions concerned with sickness, exercise and food preparation are included.

Patients with diabetes mellitus in England are very often treated by specialists. Such treatments include routine visits with dietitians.

The number of patients each dietitian sees and the short instruction time for each may make the diet instruction less than perfect but high quality instruction materials and methods were noted in visits to the classes.

Although as everywhere, the instruction varies with the clinic, counselors, and client, the English system is usually simpler than commonly used in the United States. Total kilocalories and carbohydrates are often the only nutrients considered. High sugar foods are avoided. The authors hope that such simplicity is retained even though there appears to be a move toward the more complicated fat restrictions used in the United States.

It should be noted that British food analysis data and caloric determinations may be more accurate than some of those in the U.S. because carbohydrate is determined by analysis and sugars are quoted in glucose units and calculated at 3.75 kcal per gram of glucose.[3]

REFERENCES

1. U.S. Department of Health and Human Services. *The Surgeon General's Report on Nutrition and Health*. U.S.DHHS Publication number 88-50211. Washington, D.C. 1988.

2. Dishrow, D.D.: Ambulatory nutrition care: Adults—diabetes mellitus in costs and benefits of nutrition services, a literature review, *Suppl J Am Diet Assoc* 89:4:S-35, April 1989.

3. Paul, A.A., Southgate, D.A.T.: *The Composition of Foods*, 4th revised ed. London: Her Majesty's Stationery Office, 1978.

Section IV:
Nutrition in Special Conditions

INTRODUCTION

When patients have multiple medical disorders, priority should be given to the nutritional considerations for which hospitalization is indicated. It should be emphasized that diabetes can be controlled with a variety of food plans and that no food is forbidden. Possible drug and nutrient interactions need to be addressed.

SECTION IV: CHAPTER I
THE HOSPITALIZED PATIENT

Hospital routines make the individualized treatments, recommended in other sections of this book, goals that can not be met immediately. A good dietary history may have to be postponed as must the initial diet prescription. The diet ordered for the patient with diabetes will depend on the status of the patient in regard to both diabetes and any other condition.

An estimated energy prescription should be ordered (caloric amounts calculated according to Table 1, Section I) and there should be no "standard" diabetic diet order that is used regardless of the patient's size or degree of control.

Hospitals should establish policies for admission and early diet orders. The materials used in this section are based on those developed by Easton and Blackburn for the University Hospital SUNY Stonybrook, N.Y. and used with permission. The diet orders should describe the type of diabetes and treatment (oral agents or insulin) and any modifications for age, size, condition or presence of other conditions. (See Section I, Chapters I-IV.)

Many hospitals do use Exchange List Patterns but these should not be called A.D.A. diets (see Section I, Chapter IV) and adaptation of the selective menu or some other system is often preferred when the staff becomes familiar with different plans. Some patterns of the Exchange Lists are given in Appendix VI. The lower caloric food patterns do not have fruit juice or even fruit for breakfast because of frequent morning hyperglycemia, and no meat exchange at that meal either because most patients do not want to "waste" the very limited amounts of meat allowed or there may be a cholesterol restriction.

Tables 22 and 23 give general diet advice for the hospitalized patient with diabetes according to the status of diabetes. Caution: the "listed" diet prescription in the chart or given by the patient in a history is rarely an indication of the patient's intake or the prescription needed at hospitalization.

Of course, insulin must be closely monitored for the IDDM patient in order for the food consumed to be used. Complete records of food intake should be kept. The usual so-called "calorie count" is often sufficient and familiar to hospital personnel. Patients and significant others can often complete these forms. The forms must be evaluated promptly and changes in insulin and/or food promptly made. Suggestions for discharge diets for patients with diabetes mellitus are given in Table 24.

SECTION IV: CHAPTER II
NUTRITIONAL STANDARDS AND EVALUATION

The actual nutritional needs of people have not been established, but the most commonly used standards are those of the Food and Nutrition Board of the National Research Council. The 10th edition (1989) is based upon the same definitions as previous editions but a number of changes were made.[1] Adult heights and weights of designated ages are actual medians of the U.S. population as determined by HANES II, rather than arbitrary figures. Recommended allowances are given for 19 nutrients (Vitamin K and selenium added) plus energy rather that 17 nutrients in the previous edition. Age groupings for both sexes were changed to reflect accumulation of bone mass through age 24. Energy allowances for adults are similar to those given in the previous edition but were derived by different

TABLE 22. Nutritional Recommendations for Hospital Patients with IDDM

Diabetes Classifications

IDDM Newly Diagnosed	IDDM Adjustment Out of Control	IDDM Long Standing in Control
Total Energy (kcal) Calculate energy needs. Pay particular attention to needs in hospital. Monitor left over food or vomiting episodes.	Determine usual intake, especially meal spacing, exercise and prevention of hypoglycemia. Adapt diet for hospital routine.	Adapt usual intake to hospital routine. Determine actual intake compared to caloric prescription. Monitor weight changes, fever, etc. Can use selective menu.
Carbohydrates Recommend 50-60% of total kcal as CHO. If energy needs are greater than 2400 kcal, 50-60% CHO may be too large. Increase fiber gradually.	Monitor meal spacing, check misconceptions especially specialty foods. Fruit juice serving size is crucial.	Make no changes unless needed for illness. Decrease lipids for related complications.
Proteins Calculate needed protein. Use high quality protein. Recommend 0.8 gm/kg unless renal involvement.	Check protein/foods intake. Re-educate, if necessary.	Adjust only when necessary for total energy or illness. Watch renal function constantly. 0.5 gm/kg may be necessary if renal dysfunction suspected.
Fats Fats limited in low caloric diets. Lower percentage of fats slowly to prevent increased blood triglycerides.	Check related lab values and serving sizes. Decrease saturated fat.	Check kinds of fat. Determine patient knowledge. Watch self-medication of fish oils.
Fibers Increase in low energy diets if no complications. Increased when CHO is increased. Monitor growing children, pregnant patients and those with G.I. problems.	Monitor: Possibly too much or too little.	Change only if needed for disorder. Clarify role of fiber as an adjunct treatment, not a cure.
Sodium If salt sensitive and if hypertensive, decrease sodium.	Check if salt sensitive. Changes in salt make only temporary weight changes.	Change only if indicated by sensitivity or renal problems.

TABLE 23. Nutritional Recommendations for Hospital Patients with NIDDM

Diabetes Classifications

NIDDM Newly Diagnosed (Obese) Out of Control	NIDDM Long Standing In Control
Total Energy (kcal) Usually weight loss is important. Very low energy diets may be appropriate.	Adapt to hospital routine and meal spacing. Try to determine previous intake and cut for decreased activity in hospital. Can usually use selective menu.
Carbohydrates Increase carbohydrate especially polysaccharides. With increased fiber, total kcal decreased. If protein needs are high, may need to reduce CHO to 40 to 50% of total kilocalories.	Adjust to illness. Teach about carbohydrates.
Proteins Keep protein intake at adequate minimum.	Re-educate and check possible renal function. Otherwise keep the same.
Fats Low caloric diets automatically give low fat intake although some fad diets may not. Fish and fish oils may not be appropriate.	Check kinds of fat. Be cautious about changes that hinder compliance and put stress on life style.
Fibers Low energy diets usually increase fiber but use will not cure diabetes.	Be cautious of changes unless fiber is self-prescribed. Too high intake causes flatulence. Watch for impactions.
Sodium Check for salt sensitivity. If hypertension exists, the automatic salt reduction of a low caloric diet may suffice.	Salt may make low caloric diets palatable. Decrease only if indicated.

Note: Hospitalized NIDDM patients who are not obese should usually be treated as IDDM.

methods so cannot be directly compared. The RDAs for pregnant and lactating women are now given as total allowances rather than as additions. A summary table of estimated safe and adequate daily dietary intakes has been retained for those essential vitamins and minerals for which data is insufficient to establish an RDA. The

TABLE 24. Suggestions for Discharge Diet for Patients with Diabetes Mellitus

IDDM New	IDDM Out of Control	IDDM In Control at Hospital
Determine glycemic control and weight loss previous to hospitalization. Severe IDDM patients often gain weight when adjusting insulin. Suggest Food Choice Plan or Healthy Food Choices for diet instruction.	Balance energy use with insulin and exercise. Watch for hypoglycemia and spacing of foods. HBGM may encourage too much food.	Monitor only if changes in activity or medication or excess weight gain. Watch for spacing of food post-hospital.

NIDDM New Out of Control	NIDDM Long Standing in Control
Dramatic weight loss may be needed both for physical and psychological reasons. Teach serving sizes and food preparation methods. Suggest Food Choice Plan and reasonable exercise regime.	Check weight gain due to change in activity (including sleep). Teach serving sizes.

Notes: (1) All patients should have dietary monitoring and instruction from the time of admission until discharge. (2) All diet prescriptions need to be checked at 1 and 6 month post-hospitalization. More frequently if surgery or major complication was reason for hospitalization.

electrolytes, sodium, chloride and potassium, were removed from the above listing and are now given in terms of minimum requirements.

Caution: The RDAs are based on the concept that the nutrients listed are from ordinary foods and therefore may represent other nutrients in the foods. The use of these as minimum and/or required amounts is not advised. The RDAs were established for healthy people.

There have been few if any studies of people with diabetes in relationship to absorption of and need for specific nutrients, so the assumption is probably safely made that the RDA standards are the same as for people who do not have diabetes. It should be noted that often recommendations of increased RDAs are based on low intakes in the general public rather than studies of people taking the recommended amounts.

The use of supplemental vitamins because a person has diabetes is probably not necessary and may even be ill advised. The food usually eaten by people with diabetes is nutrient dense and people with NIDDM may have ample stores of vitamins and minerals.[2]

Should a vitamin/mineral supplement be prescribed for people with diabetes mellitus? Probably not, but realistically the public/ patient pressure to be safe is so great that a low dose multiple vitamin may be a lesser evil than leaving the patient prey to public and neighbor's advice or scare techniques. (See Section VI for dietary guidelines.)

SECTION IV: CHAPTER III
SPECIAL DIETS

Many special diet regimens are empirically, not scientifically, based and they "work" because of the belief, decision making or nurturing systems. Testimonial data from medical people are often based on such beliefs and perpetuate myths which may not be as harmless as surmised. For example, the belief that orange juice is too acid for an ulcerated stomach or duodenum is false unless the condition is accompanied by achlorhydria. Normally the pH of the stomach can be as low as 1.0; orange juice has a pH of 4.5. Absences of such foods may cause an unnecessary deficiency of ascorbic acid.

A combination of restrictions must always be ranked according to the severity of the disorders. The dietary management of an acute condition must take priority over all usual general nutritive advice. Patients and caregivers alike need to understand this. It is shocking to learn that a dietitian is reluctant to give a sugar based gelatin dessert to a person with diabetes because of this sugar! More shocking is the case of a nurse's aide who gave a patient with hypoglycemia "Sweet & Low" because "that is diabetic sugar"!

The liquid diet menus which follow are not adequate nutritionally and even the full liquid should be given only as long as absolutely necessary. Use of such diets are frightening to patients and family alike. Both written and oral explanations are needed.

SECTION IV: CHAPTER IV
LIQUID DIETS

Determination of Daily Base-line Fluid Requirements

	ml/kg/day
First 10 kilograms of body weight	100
Second 10 kilograms of body weight	50
All weight above 20 kilograms	20 if less than 50 years old
	15 if over 50 years old

This formula applies to all patients except infants weighing less than 5 kg and patients with massive trauma, dehydration or pathological fluid retaining states. The calculations are based on ''ideal body weight'' for height, sex, and age for obese patients, and on actual body weight for others.[3]

Clear Liquid Moderate Protein Diet

The purpose of this diet is to supply moderate levels of protein in the face of physical trauma in order to maintain or restore positive nitrogen balance. This dietary regimen requires minimal digestion. It also provides essential fat and amino acids. Candidates for this type of diet might be patients with depleted protein stores.

This diet approximates the metabolic requirement for protein and calories but does NOT meet the recommended dietary allowances for vitamins and minerals. As with all clear liquid diets, the length of use should be minimized and progressive steps taken to return the patient to a normal food intake.

Food Allowed:

Beverages	Clear tea, black coffee, decaffeinated coffee, carbonated beverage
Juices	Apple, grape or cranberry
Soups	Clear broths or bouillon
Desserts	Plain flavored gelatin, water ices
Supplements	Vivonex HN, Ensure, Vipep, etc.

Suggested Meal Pattern for Clear Liquid Diet,
Breakfast, Lunch, and Dinner

	Carbohydrate (gm)	Kcal
1 c juice	30	120
1 c gelatin made with Vivonex HN, Citrotein, etc.	60	300
1c clear broth or bouillon, coffee or tea with 2 tsp. sugar	8	30
Nourishments three times per day: 8 oz Vivonex HN, Citrotein, Vipep, etc.	60	300
Total for all 3 meals and 3 nourishments	474	2250

Clear Liquid Diet (Ordinary Foods)

	Carbohydrate (gm)	Kcal
Meal One:		
1 c apple juice	29	116
3/4 c regular, sweetened gelatin desert	30	120
Black coffee or tea with 2 tsp sugar	8	32
Meal Total	(102)	(423)
Meal Two:		
1 c apple juice	29	116
Meal Three:		
12 oz regular gingerale	29	113
1 c clear broth	5	39
1/2 c water ice	31	123
Black coffee or tea with 2 tsp sugar	8	32
Meat Total	(102)	(427)

Meal Four:		
3/4 c regular gelatin	30	120

Meal Five:		
1 c apple juice	29	116
1 c clear broth	5	39
3/4 c regular gelatin	30	120
coffee or tea with 2 tsp sugar	8	32
Meal Total	(72)	(307)

Meal Six:		
1 c grape juice	40	160

Total for Six Meals	(311)	(1278)

Full Liquid Diet

The full liquid diet more closely approaches nutrient adequacy and can be calculated to meet the RDAs. However, the volume of foods necessary and dislike of some items make adequacy less likely. The definition of liquid varies with institutions and professionals. Eggs and baked custards may not be included in some plans.

Sample Menu-Day One

	Carbohydrate (gm)	Kcal
Meal One:		
1 pkg Carnation instant breakfast	23	130
(1 c 2% low fat milk)	12	121
1/2 c regular plain oatmeal	13	72
1/4 c regular applesauce	13	49
coffee or tea		
Total Meal	(61)	(372)

Meal Two:

1 c cream of mushroom soup w/milk	15	203
3/4 c regular gelatin	30	120
1/2 c regular baked custard	15	153
coffee or tea		
Total Meal	(61)	(372)

Meal Three:

1 c grape juice	40	160
1 c cream of potato soup w/milk	17	148
2 soft scrambled eggs	2	158
3/4 c vanilla ice cream	24	202
coffee or tea		
Meal Total	(83)	(668)

Meal Four:

3/4 c regular gelatin	30	120
1 c 2% lowfat milk	12	121
3/4 c regular strained oatmeal	20	108
Meal Total	(62)	(349)

Total for Four Meals	(266)	(1865)

Sample Menu - Day Two

	Carbohydrate gm	Kcal
Meal One:		
1/2 c grape juice	20	80
1 pkg instant oatmeal with maple syrup		
&brown sugar	32	163
1 c 2% lowfat milk	12	121
coffee or tea		
Meal Total	(64)	(364)
Meal Two:		
1/2 c peach nectar	17	67
1/2 c creamed cottage cheese — 2% fat	3	117

2/3 c regular tapioca	18	116
1 c 2% lowfat milk	12	112
1 banana pudding pop	16	94
coffee or tea		
Meal Total	(66)	(364)
Meal Three:		
1/2 c regular cranberry juice	19	74
1 c cream of chicken soup with milk	9	116
1 c lowfat vanilla yogurt	31	194
2 soft scrambled eggs	2	223
1/2 c 2% lowfat milk	6	60
Meal Total	(67)	(667)
Meal Four:		
1 c regular pasteurized eggnog	35	342
Total for Four Meals	(232)	(1879)

SECTION IV: CHAPTER V
FAT CONTROLLED DIETS

Diets used for people with NIDDM and some IDDM are often very low in total fat because of the need to decrease total energy (calories). The polyunsaturated to saturated fat ratio (See Glossary) can be increased with use of oils instead of fats (caution: some oils are still high in saturated fats such as coconut, palm, or other oils) and soft margarine. The polyunsaturated to saturated fat ratio in very low fat diets may only be of academic interest and should not be a priority if it is only a preventative measure without laboratory values or genetic history supporting these measures.

Some patients with hyperlipoproteinemia may improve their blood profiles with dietary manipulation. The usefulness of this is under dispute but may be advised for the patient who has had a heart attack or has strong familial tendencies toward hyperlipoproteinemia.

The reduction of cholesterol in diets of people with diabetes is also one that may be questioned because it may lead to a severe restriction of eggs. Eggs are a low fat, reasonably inexpensive source of high quality protein and therefore restrictions should not be necessary unless the blood cholesterol levels are elevated.

The highly unsaturated fatty acids from fish (omega-3) have been receiving considerable attention regarding their possible favorable effect on blood lipids. However, the understanding of the role of omega-6 (N-6) and omega-3 (N-3) (Glossary) polyunsaturated fatty acids is far from complete and supplementary use of fish oils should not be encouraged.[4] The use of fish (broiled, steamed or baked) as an entre 2-5 times a week is beneficial in some people.

Low fat diets (40-45 grams) may be achieved with the use of skim milk, low fat cheeses, low fat meats (boiled, baked or broiled with skin and visible fat removed), no biscuits, doughnuts, pancakes, waffles, fats removed from soups and plain vegetables cooked or raw. Desserts made with pastries, toppings, creams and so forth must be avoided. A low cholesterol diet is achieved using the above measures and by limiting the use of eggs, number and size of servings of even low fat meats and fishes.

High fiber diets have been used with some success in the management of hyperlipoproteinemia. It should be noted that all diets for hyperlipoproteinemia are of the patterns given above. When triglycerides are elevated the carbohydrate portion of the diet is limited to less than 45% of calories. The lipid picture is constantly changing and the treatment of hyperlipoproteinemia by diet is very complicated. Prevention is probably best served with weight control and limiting of total fat.

SECTION IV: CHAPTER VI
DIETS IN RENAL FAILURE

The diet for a person on dialysis requires much understanding, planning and education. Advice and monitoring by a renal dietitian is essential. The information given here is general and should be considered preliminary to appropriate dietary counseling.

The restriction of protein varies according to the degree of nitrogen retention and renal condition. The amount of protein prescribed may be limited in some cases to 0.5 gm per kilogram of body weight.[5] Food proteins should be of high quality (high biological value). The use of very low protein diets is questioned by some in terms of the upset of metabolic base.[6]

With a restricted protein diet, sufficient energy from carbohydrate and fat is needed so that proteins from both food and body tissues are not used for energy. Calories may range from 25 to 45 kcal per kg body weight depending on the degree of catabolism. It is usually necessary to add sugar (if tolerated) to increase energy intake. This often needs careful explanation[6] for the person who has been on traditional diets. With the new exchange list allotment of 3 gm of protein for 1 bread or cereal exchange, it is possible that miscalculation of protein could occur for the actual foods used.

The limitation of fluids is often very difficult especially in hot weather and subtropical climates. The patient may find use of candies and sugars increase thirst. Less sweet sugars such as lactose (if tolerated) may be used.

SECTION IV: CHAPTER VII
ELECTROLYTE BALANCE – IMBALANCE

Charts giving sodium and potassium values are readily available. Often indigenous or culturally preferred foods are not included. If the sodium or potassium value is left blank, it means that the amount is unknown, not that the electrolyte does not exist in the food. For example, mango season in Florida often triggers excess potassium loads.

"Non-productive" sources of sodium such as water or medicines are often not considered. (See Low Sodium Diets.)

Sodium Modified Diets

Diet Principles

Because of the role of sodium in water balance, dietary sodium is restricted whenever a patient retains fluids. Therefore, a sodium restricted diet is recommended in the presence of edema, kidney and liver disorders, congestive heart failure, hypertension, toxemia of pregnancy, and whenever sodium-retaining drugs such as cortisone and ACTH are used.

Common daily adult intakes of sodium range rather widely according to habit from about 4 to 6 gm per day.[7] The main source of dietary sodium is common table salt and to a lesser extent baking soda and baking powder. Most salt substitutes and low sodium baking powder contain increased amounts of potassium to replace the sodium. Salt contains 2300 mg of sodium per teaspoon, and baking soda contains 1000 mg of sodium per teaspoon.

Moderate sodium restriction can be effected with the use of no added salt or restriction of high salt foods. Even restricting total amounts of foods greatly reduces sodium intake.

Almost all foods contain sodium and a high intake of food can mean an increased sodium intake even with no restricted foods included. Conversely, restricted food intake may mean a very low sodium intake. Multiple restrictions are conflicting and severe restriction may mean that food intake is seriously affected.

Ordering the Diet

Three levels of sodium may be specified depending on the severity of the patient's symptoms. The diet must be specifically ordered by amounts of sodium.

2000-3000 mg sodium 85-130 mEq	MILD restriction. No added salt. Eliminates all salty foods and the salt shaker.
1000 mg sodium 45 mEq	MODERATE restriction. All foods are prepared without salt.
500 mg sodium 20 mEq	SEVERE restriction. Limits milk, meat bread and certain vegetables. All food prepared without salt.

Potassium Modified Diets

Diet Principles

Potassium depletion can occur during prolonged intravenous feeding, after severe diarrhea, during diabetic acidosis, and in patients receiving diuretics. If alkalosis occurs with the potassium depletion, additional chloride must be provided also.

In the acute phase, potassium chloride preparations may be

given. In chronic conditions, as when diuretic treatment is on a long term basis, adequate replacement should be achieved through food.

With NIDDM individuals on caloric restricted diets, a potassium supplement is often indicated. Attempting to consume an adequate potassium intake will often increase their energy intake and/or blood glucose particularly when they use bananas and other high potassium fruits. Some vegetables are high in potassium (see list below) and might be suggested to replace bananas.

If the diet is restricted in sodium, and a salt substitute containing potassium salts is used, this will supply approximately 600 mg (15 mEq) potassium per half teaspoonful. Low sodium fresh milk prepared by ion exchange provides approximately 600 mg (15 mEq) potassium per cup. Low sodium baking powders are also high in potassium.

High Potassium Foods

Each serving of the following foods provides approximately 600 mg of potassium. These foods can be used liberally, especially immediately after ingestion of diuretics, if consideration is given to the total caloric level of the regular food intake pattern.

Apricots, dried 4 (8 halves)	Peaches, 2 large fresh
Avocado 1/2	Pear 1 large raw
Almonds 1/2 cup	Peanuts 1/3 cup
Banana 1 medium	Potato 1 small baked
Cantaloupe 1/2 medium	Prunes or plums 3
Dates 1/2 cup	Prune juice 1 cup
French fries 1/2 cup	Pumpkin 1 cup canned
Grapefruit juice 1 1/2 cup	Tomato 1 large raw
Molasses 3 Tablespoons	Tomato juice 1 cup
Oranges 2 medium	Walnuts 1/2 cup
Pineapple juice 1 1/2 cup	Wheat germ 1/3 cup

Conversion: 39 mg potassium = 1 mEq
          23 mg sodium = 1 mEq

For people with diabetes the caloric content of fruit make choices of vegetables useful.

SECTION IV: CHAPTER VIII
GASTROINTESTINAL DISORDERS

The classic saying "If a patient says something doesn't agree with him, it doesn't" applies especially to gastrointestinal tract conditions. Many people have devised an acceptable dietary plan that excludes foods that are disliked or not tolerated. Radical changes in food ingested may be upsetting both psychologically and physically. Lactose deficiency is well known but less is known about the decreased secretion of other digestive enzymes if not used. Regeneration of the enzymes if it occurs may take up to a month. Flatulence often occurs in these diets as increased sucrose is introduced after a long abstinence. The liquid diets that are high in sucrose may be a case in point.

The conservative treatment for hiatal hernia includes small frequent meals taken in an upright position. Acids and irritants such as spices and coffee can cause distress. Glucose monitoring and carefully scheduled meals can make management of hiatal hernia and diabetes possible. The prescription needs to be individualized and monitored by a dietitian.

Ulcers, gastric and/or duodenal (in the presence of acid), require medical control. This may include beta-blocking agents and antacids.

The traditional bland diet has long been contraindicated in all of its forms (Sippy, conservative bland, soft bland, etc.). The basis for foods on these diets was pragmatic and was preferable to starvation. Milk and cream do stimulate acid production and frequent feedings increase acid production. Ground foods, toasted bread, and lukewarm foods all are antiquated treatments. These should only be recommended if they are in the folklore and historical experience of the patient. The trauma resolved in any treatment may be too severe to be worth the change.

The only known effect and documented irritants are the peppers, black, red, and white. Fried foods may have satiety value but may cause gastric distress probably not related to the ulcer. The use of coffee or decaffeinated coffees have also been found to be irritating. Alcohol and cigarettes are also irritants.

Gastroparesis diabeticorum, the gastric manifestation of diabetic autonomic neuropathy is thought to occur in 20 to 30 percent of persons with diabetes mellitus.[8] Persons with gastroparesis should be cautioned against the use of high fiber diets.[9] (See Section VI, Chapter VI.)

Many myths surround low residue or non-residue diets. Residue occurs even in the G.I. tract from the sloughing off of cells. Milk and wheat products do produce a residue. The pureeing of vegetables or grinding of meats does not remove the residual fibers. Low residue diets are now rarely used for treatment of diverticulosis as it may trigger the formation of diverticulitis. True low residue diets should not include use of food irritants. Use strained fruits and vegetables, tender, lightly cooked non-fibrous meats and fats, and avoid seeds, nuts, whole grains, and other sources of non-digestible materials. Although sugars do not contain fiber, they may encourage gas formation. During diarrhea and chronic intestinal diseases much energy is lost from the fact that foods are not absorbed.

The beliefs of faddists and quacks have been involved in the diagnosis of allergic reactions to common food and non-food substances. This is usually "supported" by a series of laboratory analyses called "cytotoxic testing" (see Glossary). Although true food allergies do exist and therefore, the offending foods should be avoided, allergic reactions as diagnosed by cytotoxic and other spurious methods are not true ones and therefore the "cure" does not exist either. Palliative measures such as catering to such diagnoses are dangerous for the gullible and may result in a nutrient deficient diet and possible spreading of ignorance and quackery. The food supply is so abundant in the United States that patients can be taught to avoid true food allergies in their diets. Reputable medical personnel need to be aware of quackery in the community.

SECTION IV: CHAPTER IX
CANCER

The current recommendation concerning possible protection from cancer, i.e., high fiber, low saturated fats, are easily incorporated into the dietary choices of people with diabetes. A reliable "anti-cancer diet" is still not available.[10] For the most part coding a dietary treatment "protective" against cancer is misleading (most evidence is from animals) because the evidence from animals suggests that protection against cancer translates as reduced risk.[10]

The use of glucose monitoring is essential if the patient is undergoing treatment for cancer. Energy from any source is important and sugar may or may not be tolerated. Decreased senses of taste and smell as well as decreased saliva accompany chemotherapy and some head and neck cancers. Many people find meals unappealing and therefore high caloric food is encouraged. High fiber and low caloric liquids usually must be decreased because of the patient's limited desire for food and the necessity for all possible energy to be consumed.

Chemotherapy treatments ideally are scheduled at the patient's "off eating" times. If a patient eats a good breakfast, therapy should probably be scheduled later in the day. Insulin should also be adjusted to the patient's eating time and incidence of nausea.

Supplemental foods such as puddings and high caloric drinks may be used but the commercial preparations are often expensive and are not well accepted. It should be noted that between meal supplements may decrease consumption at meals. The careful use of ordinary foods with added butter, sugar, cream, and so on may be preferable. Again, it may be necessary to teach patients and caregivers alike that traditionally limited foods are often advisable during treatment for cancer.

SECTION IV: CHAPTER X
DRUG–NUTRIENT INTERACTIONS

Drugs used to prevent or treat disease, have a variety of interactions with nutrients. The person with diabetes needs to know when these interactions may be dangerous in terms of diabetes treatment and control or health in general.[7] The effects of specific medications on blood glucose require the attention of physicians and pharmacists. The most important concern for the dietary counselor is that food intake is not "blamed" for all glucose excursions even though some adjustments in food intake may be necessary.

There are two major concerns regarding the interaction of drugs and nutrients: (1) the effect of drugs on the nutritional status of the individual and (2) the effect of nutrients and nutritional status on the absorption and metabolism of drugs.

Drugs can affect nutritional status by causing an alteration in food intake by increasing or decreasing appetite, alteration of taste or smell of food or by causing nausea and/or vomiting. Drugs can also alter the absorption of nutrients by changing the motility of the gastrointestinal tract, by changing bile activity or by the formation of drug-nutrient complexes. Drugs can also cause the inactivation of digestive enzymes or can cause damage to the mucosal cells in the G.I. tract causing alteration of nutrient absorption. Drugs can also alter the metabolism and utilization of nutrients as well as their excretion.

Nutrients and nutritional status can effect the absorption and metabolism of drugs. Drug metabolism is altered in states of nutritional deficiency. It is also influenced by the rate of intestinal absorption, the presence of other diseases, liver function, concomitant administration of other drugs or by the interaction of the drug and a food constituent. Other mechanisms by which food components alter drug therapy are in the distribution of the drug in the body, the metabolism of the drug and the mechanism of excretion of the drug.

Absorption of many drugs from the gastrointestinal tract is affected by the presence of food. Generally drugs are absorbed more slowly when food is present which can either cause a decrease in the drug dose by not achieving effective blood levels or the slow absorption can act as a sustained release prolonging the effect of the drug. Most drugs affected by the presence of food will carry a warning to take with food, or take on an empty stomach. Alcohol can affect the absorption or metabolism of drugs. Large doses of alcohol inhibit some hepatic enzymes and thus decrease drug metabolism or can increase the toxic side effects of some drugs.[11] In patients taking sulfonylurea compounds, alcohol inhibits enzymes necessary for hepatic gluconeogenesis thus enhancing the hypoglycemic effect of the drug.[7]

People who take multiple drugs and for extended periods of time are those who are likely to be most affected by drug-nutritional interactions.[7] Elderly people are most likely to be in this group.

The complexity of the diet components and of drug responses makes the clinical implications of interactions complex and many times hard to predict. The diet counselor and physician should help the patient change food patterns to minimize the interaction effects.

The list of nutrient-drug interactions is increasing rapidly but the significance of such interactions is hard to validate because of variables such as the quantity of drug or nutrient involved, the presence of disease conditions and the age, size and general physical condition of the patient. The probability of the occurrence and the clinical significance of any interaction has to be evaluated in the individual patient rather than by using generalized rules.

For patients with diabetes mellitus, drugs which influence appetite directly affect the ability to comply with food prescriptions. Some drugs alter the absorption of nutrients while some food components (e.g., fiber) limit the absorption of some drugs. A change in the transit time in the G.I. tract (usually by the use of laxatives) can alter the absorption of both drugs and nutrients. Antacids change the acidity of the stomach and may interfere with drugs that need an acid environment for absorption. Patients should be made aware of the possible nutrient-drug interactions that occur with over-the-counter preparations they may be taking as well as with their prescription drugs.

Counselors need to take a detailed inventory of a patient's prescription and non-prescription drug intake. Information on specific prescription drugs and over-the-counter medications are available in several publications and from the manufacturers of the products.

A common concern for people with diabetes is the sugar content of both prescribed and over-the-counter medications. The diet counselor needs to ascertain if these are taken in sufficient amounts to increase the level of sugar in the diet pattern. The patient needs to understand that "sugar free" is not necessarily non-caloric. The patient needs to learn how to read labels and how to judge if the amount of sugar is significant. Many sugar free medications are marketed[12] but they may not be necessary for the occasional, moderate user of ordinary medications.

Nutrient supplements containing massive doses are sometimes used. They may be prescribed by the physician or self-prescribed. When nutrients are taken in large amounts they are considered drugs and side effects or other interactions can occur. The patient's medical supervisor should ascertain whether the patient is following some dangerous practice with the self-prescription of supplements.

REFERENCES

1. Food and Nutrition Board, National Research Council: *Recommended Dietary Allowances*. 10th revised ed.: Washington, D.C., National Academy of Sciences, 1989.

2. Beaton, G.H.: Criteria of an adequate diet. Chapter 35. In *Modern Nutrition in Health and Disease* 7th ed. by Shils, M.E. and Young, V.R.: Lea and Febiger: Philadelphia, 1988.

3. Souba, W.W. and Wilmer, D.W.: Diet and nutrition in the care of the patient with surgery, trauma and sepsis. Chapt 62. in *Modern Nutrition in Health and Disease* 7th ed. by Shils, M.E. and Young, V.R.: Lea and Febiger: Philadelphia, 1988.

4. Sousky, A. and Raobbins, D.C.: Fish oils the net effect. *Diabetes Care* 12:4:302, Apr 1989.

5. Cearcella A., DiMizio, G., Stefoni, S., Borgnino, L.C., Vanni, P.: Reduced albuminuria after dietary protein restriction in insulin-dependent diabetic patients with clinical nephrophophy. *Diabetes Care* 10:407, 1987.

6. Brodsky, I.G., Robbins, D.C.: Editorial: Safety of low-protein diets where's the beef. *Diabetes Care* 12:6:435, June 1989.

7. *The Surgeon General's Report on Nutrition and Health*. U.S. Dept of Health and Human Services. DHHS Publ. No. (PHS)88-50210, 1988.

8. Canivet, B., Greiss, G., Freygy, P., and Dagey, X.:Fibre diabetes and risk of bezoar. *Lancet* 2:862, Oct 1980.

9. Emerson, A.P.: Foods high in fiber and phytobezoar formation. *J Am Diet Assoc* 87:12:1675, Dec 1987.

10. Newsbreaks: "Anti-Cancer diet" needs additional study. *Nutrition Today* 23:6:5, Nov/Dec 1988.

11. Rubin, E., Gang, H., Misra, P.S., and Lieber, C.S.: Inhibition of drug metabolism by acute ethanol intoxication: A hepatic microsomal mechanism. *Am J Med* 49:801, 1970.

12. Dunlop, L., Pruitt, B., Campbell, R.K.: Sugar-free preparations by therapeutic category. *The Diabetes Educator* 15:3:226 May/Jun 1989.

Section V:
Weight Correction and Control

INTRODUCTION

The most common and often most difficult problem in treating the patient with NIDDM is accompanying obesity. The patient is usually female, often sedentary and middle aged. This chapter is designed to present primarily the problems of this group and some suggestions for treatment. The terms "correction" and "control" are both important because the strategies used effectively in correction may be abandoned in the long-term control period.

The proliferation of weight reduction diets has been so great for years that the word "diet" has come to mean weight loss itself. It is important for health team members to be aware of the public concern with weight and weight reduction and help patients benefit from this concern.

SECTION V: CHAPTER I
WEIGHT CORRECTION

Weight correction and control has become important with IDDM patients who are on tight control regimes. Some of the information in this chapter is useful for this group but a better solution is probably a decrease in food rather than an increase in insulin to control hyperglycemia.[1]

Although weight counseling is usually used to mean weight reduction, achievement of appropriate body weight may mean an increase in weight for some people with diabetes. This is often the case with newly diagnosed IDDM patients who have not utilized food energy because of lack of insulin or people who have used insufficient insulin. Patient induced ketosis is a method of effecting weight control and has been defined in this book as diabetic bulimia (see Glossary). Patients should be observed to determine if this is intentionally or even accidently occurring.

Hunger or learned symptoms of hypoglycemia may also encourage improper food consumption or the increase and/or delayed insulin production in NIDDM diabetes may account for patients never feeling full or always being hungry. The current recommendations to only eat when hungry or to simply "cut down" probably are nonproductive for the obese patient. Appetite control for them must be a learned activity and will take external or deliberate personal control for years, perhaps forever. Use of behavior modification techniques are recommended. Avoidance of "all you can eat" meals and salad bars may be necessary until such control is learned.

The formation of water with the oxidation of fat is often not considered in weight loss. This water can be retained in the body for some time allowing for a plateau or even weight gain. Expecting this to happen may help a patient on a weight control regime to continue. Another force, often temporary, is the decrease in salt, either from the type of foods and food preparation on the weight correction diet, intermittent salt restriction or just a decreased food intake. If the patient understands that weight fluctuations are normal, then weight changes measured at frequent intervals should not be alarming. Body weight is usually lowest early in the morning. Daily or every other day weighing may be appropriate.

The adaptation of the body to starvation whether self-imposed or not is a well known but sometimes ignored phenomenon. The basal metabolic rate decreases during starvation and consequently weight loss may not occur even with decreased energy intakes. The time this takes may be from 3 to 6 weeks but may occur more quickly in frequent starvers.

Fasting as a weight modification system has long been used and often deplored by medical personnel especially dietitians. Diets contributing less than 800 to 1000 calories are not considered to be adequate nutritionally. However, the first goal of diet therapy is to treat the disorder and short term or intermittent fasts may be effective in NIDDM. Obese people usually have large stores of fat soluble vitamins. Water soluble vitamins such as ascorbic acid are in the body water which in effect is a storage (saturation) which may prevent any deficiency symptoms for several months. Protein cannot be stored and authorities vary from advocating high quality protein to prevent tissue loss to stating that any protein in a hypocaloric diet will be used as energy. Careful medical monitoring of very low caloric diets is essential.[2]

The advantages of fasting are the removal of the patient from usual food concerned activities. Complete fasts (3 days is a common time) may be more effective than low calorie diets for this purpose. The occurrence of ketosis decreases the appetite and if properly controlled may not be dangerous. Headaches, dry mouth (even with water allowed) and constipation often accompany fasts. Patients may experience a "high" in activity or become lethargic both intermittently. These conditions require physical and psychological monitoring.

The foods used during fasting may be only liquids, formula diets, or carefully chosen small servings of ordinary foods. Note: a diet less than 800 calories may be necessary for a small, elderly, obese female for any weight loss to occur where a 1000 calorie diet may actually be a fasting regimen for a tall, active male. Some liquid diet programs are reviewed in Section IV, Chapter IV.

SECTION V: CHAPTER II
WEIGHT LOSS TECHNIQUES

It is important that health professionals treating patients with diabetes be alerted to the weight loss programs that are currently popular and how their patient can be effected.

The fad diets concerned with uneven intakes such as the "Rotation Diet" can be adapted if weight loss only is desired. Diets recommending a high fat, low carbohydrate intake such as "Adkins and Stillman Diets" are not advised for treatment of diabetes. The one food and food group diets such as "The Beverly Hills Diet" and "Food for Life Diets" need to be carefully critiqued. Diets recommending high potency supplements may be dangerous. None of these diets is recommended for the patient with IDDM even if weight loss is desired. The use of "special menus," as described below and found in Appendix VII, may be useful or a "new" system such as the Food Choice Plan makes use of some of the attractions of fad diets without some of the dangers.

A preplanned menu for a period of days or even weeks is an attractive method of weight control for some people. Some menus with various names and compositions are often passed from person to person. The discipline may be useful and the menus may be adequate. Usually, they are some form of high fat/low carbohydrate meals which initiate rapid weight loss (water loss) and are high in satiety value. Often they are so unattractive or deficient or expensive that the person soon tires of them.

The "special menus" (Appendix VII) utilize differing strategies and mealtimes.

Special Menu I: Menus for three days with two meals each with approximately 800 kcal/day. Relatively high in fiber, low in fat, and can be low in sodium if sodium is limited in preparation. The eating times should be held or even extended to 10 A.M. to 6 P.M. This utilizes the often repeated condition of "I don't get hungry until I eat." Note: These are low in nutrients from milk and may be low in iron for women. No fruit juice is allowed and only small amounts of low sugar fruits are permitted.

Special Menu II: Three days of three meals using some convenience foods to allow for less food preparation, reduced appetite and temptation. No fruit juices are included and menus are relatively low in calcium and riboflavin.

Special Menu III: Three days of menus 1200-1500 kcal each, using all restaurant and fast foods (some brand names are included but substitutes are acceptable if equal in kilocalories). These menus are high sodium and fat because of food preparation methods used in fast food restaurants. Note: Eggs are used frequently because of patients who have reported reluctance to eat only cereal. (Several patients have reported that they cannot eat meals with business contacts unless this type is allowed). Before and after meals glucose monitoring might be very useful on any of these diets to see if any meal causes a glucose excursion.

The conditions and changing moods accompanying weight reduction diets are important to the health care providers. Some of these and possible remedies are detailed in Table 25.

TABLE 25. Conditions Occurring During Weight Correction Regimens in Patients with NIDDM

1. No Weight Loss (or Minimal) after Initial Water Balance Correction

Effect	Possible Cause(s)	Possible Remedies
Stress, feeling of failure	Lack of understanding of regimen.	Repeat and monitor instruction.
	Reluctance to accept responsibility.	Work with patient to determine food intake.
Professionals, family, and friends doubt patient's honesty and commitment.	Recalculate energy needs and use. Formula may be high for actual patient.	Check patient's ideas of serving sizes, menus, food patterns.
	Actual knowledge and intake different from calculated.	Look for large intakes of food effecting energy intake, decrease in energy use.
		Look for specific foods that may be higher than calculated, ex. use of higher fat milk, higher fat meats.
		Look for non-food items, ex. cough drops/syrup, gum. Look for large intakes of foods, ex. salads/salad dressing.
Hypoglycemic agents may be given.	Weight gain may occur with improved glucose utilization.	Reemphasize that diet is still a needed treatment and increase diet related checkups and instruction.
	Increased hunger, fear of hypoglycemia and increased number of meals.	Encourage decrease or discontinuing hypoglycemic agents if condition allows
		Recalculate diet prescription and add night meal if necessary.

TABLE 25 (continued)

2. Plateau Following Acceptable or Rapid Weight Loss

Effect	Possible Cause(s)	Possible Remedies
Patient becomes discouraged and may discontinue diet control efforts.	Change in size or adaptation to starvation.	Recalculate diet prescription or increase exercise.
	Decrease in energy use.	Use of different foods which need to be calculated, recheck serving sizes and food items, "hidden" calories, change diet plan/system.
	Familiarity has decreased accuracy.	

SECTION V: CHAPTER III
BEHAVIOR MODIFICATION

Changes in any dietary pattern or regimen involve behavior modification. The term is usually used to represent some stylized behaviors prescribed for weight control regimens. The value of these behaviors varies with the patient and the usefulness varies with the commitment and lifestyle of the patient. Early behavior changes may affect weight loss even if they are not useful in the long term. The usual behavior modifications are listed in Table 26 with signs indicating possible short-term and long-term usefulness. Weight reduction is easier for some people with complete or nearly complete lifestyle changes. In these instances all or most of the behaviors may be useful. For long-term adaptation to reduced food intake, emphasis may be better placed on the most used behaviors which are listed with + + + +. (See Table 26.)

Determination of the most productive behavior change is relatively time consuming. One way to simplify this is to have detailed records kept prior to the conference. These records should include foods eaten (amounts are very important), times of meals, places, and feelings about foods and meals.

TABLE 26. Behaviors for Weight Control and Correction

Purpose of Behaviors*	Probable Effectiveness for NIDDM Patients
A. To control amount of food	
1. Recording food intake (short term)	1. ++++
2. Watching portion sizes	2. ++++
3. Removing serving dishes from table	3. ++++
4. Using smaller plates	4. ++++
5. Leaving food on plate	5. ++++
6. Avoiding second helpings	6. ++++
7. Putting utensil down between bites	7. ++
8. Counting bites and "chews"	8. ++
9. If reading glasses are used, wear them while eating	9. ++++
B. To decrease food cues that condition eating behaviors	
1. Eating in only one place	1. +
2. Substituting other social activities	2. ++
3. No other activity when eating (i.e. watching T.V.)	3. ++
4. Mid-meal meandering	4. +++
5. Getting up when finished	5. +++
C. Controlling food available and nutrient content	
1. Reading food labels	1. ++++
2. Modifying preparation	2. ++++
3. Modifying recipes	3. ++
4. Shopping with a list	4. +
5. Shopping after meals	5. ++
6. Using prepared foods	6. +++
7. Keep food out of sight or not in home	7. ++
8. Preplanning meals	8. ++++
9. Choosing food ahead of function	9. ++++
D. Behaviors to increase energy use	
1. Increasing walking	1. ++++
2. Increase other forms of exercise	2. +++
3. Decreasing sleep or reclining time	3. ++++
4. Increasing non-food related activities	4. +++

* Caution: There are more behaviors listed than can be used all at once.

Using a record, the diet counselor and the patient together can determine which behaviors can and should be changed. It is easy to say that patients are stubborn or resist change; this is often not so. Foods and eating behaviors are changing constantly with the use of new brands, going to new restaurants, trying new recipes, and addition or loss of friends, to name only a few. Determining changes can be productive for control of diabetes. The goal of lowering of blood glucose may seem to be one of little importance in terms of life stresses and social needs. For example, insisting that a person eat at a table without the television may really be a foolish behavior on which to focus while insisting on wearing glasses while measuring food may be an important one.

SECTION V: CHAPTER IV
COMMERCIAL PROGRAMS FOR WEIGHT LOSS

There are many commercial or public weight loss programs. Some are non-profit groups, some supported by agencies which sell materials, services and/or food. The quality of these programs depends on the quality of the directors and leaders. Some chains or national programs have exceptionally fine scientists developing the materials and products only to have lay leaders who are "successes" dilute or misinterpret the information at the local level. Support groups of people with diabetes (hospital sponsored) might be preferred. Caution: Information given or exchanged about diabetes in all groups should be carefully monitored.

Some people lose weight with the help of these programs, and they enjoy the fellowship and the reinforcement. The medical professional must see that the advice is not harmful, the cost not prohibitive, and correct or clarify misconceptions that arise (see counseling strategies, Section I, Chapter III).

Popular Weight Loss Techniques

People with diabetes are not isolated from society in general and weight loss programs are popularized in all media.

Sometimes these diets are passed from hand to hand or by word of mouth. The so-called "Mayo Clinic Diet" is an example of this method of instruction. It is also called the Grapefruit Diet, and the Egg Diet. The incorrect information given about the effect of grapefruit on weight loss is "known" by more people than correct information.

These regimens range from reasonable to bizarre, from deceptively simple and practical to actually dangerous. If any one of these fads were "the answer" that it claims to be, all of the others would be obsolete. Keeping up with these diets is difficult. The radio, television and even newspapers may interview the authors and followers as actual news and thereby give credibility to the fad. Some media programs will use credible authorities to debate the authors or refute the rationale.

The description of program types listed below are meant to give the health professional some information and ways to aid patients. The need for people with NIDDM to find an effective weight loss program is often crucial to adequate care. The often quoted advice of "gradual weight loss on an adequate diet" may be impossible advice for them to follow. Some of the descriptions and all of the cost figures are from an article in Changing Times.[3]

1. Formula/liquid diets—Physician supervised: Optifast is the most commonly known program but there are others that are similar and require medical supervision and repeated visits. The approximate cost is $2500-3000[3] for six months with an additional $500 charge for a six month maintenance period after goal weight is reached.

The advantages of such programs for people with diabetes are that (1) the information would be adapted for them; (2) weight loss is rapid and may allow for reduced medications and (3) patients have a program that removes them from food temptations and is socially acceptable.

The disadvantages are that (1) patients may regain weight and become "addicted" to formulas for weight control rather than just correction; (2) the diets are nutritionally questionable and should not be extended for long periods and (3) there are side effects.

2. Strictly commercial/over-the-counter: Many of these powdered formulas such as the Cambridge Diet have gone out of busi-

ness or at least, favor as their (lack of) efficacy or actual client harm has been documented. Some products (such as Slim Fast) are still readily available and may recommend use for only one or two meals a day.

Such plans for a person with diabetes need careful professional scrutiny.

3. Food plans such as Nutri/System: The companies provide food in preportioned packages. The cost is relatively high, $300-400 for a weight loss of 40 pounds[3] plus $50/week for the food. The foods are sweetened with "Nutri-Sweet"[3] and are found by some to accomplish weight loss because of poor palatability. This system may be useful for some patients if the menus are reviewed for adequacy and medical monitoring continued.

4. Private counselling: Registered dietitians give private individual and group counselling as do clinics and other groups such as universities. The important factor for people with diabetes is that they know their disease and prescription well and that the advice be compatible with that of the medical supervisor.

Nutritionists may or may not be dietitians (see Glossary) and patients should be cautioned to find out the credentials of people using this title.

5. Some chains such as "Diet Centers"[3] give a highly structured approach and also sell vitamin/protein/mineral supplements. These should be viewed with skepticism especially when categories of foods such as dairy products are not advised.[3] The cost runs from $450-600 for a weight loss of 25 lbs.[3]

6. Books, pamphlets and celebrity programs: The short lives of these books and pamphlets indicate their questionable value. Some have impossible or expensive combinations of foods and/or inaccurate physiological reasons for efficacy. For example, one of the more recent ones, The T Factor Diet, while having some good advice about lower fat intake, states that only fat (in foods) can cause fat to be formed in the body.

The plans such as the Beverly Hills Diets that advise "flushing out the body" are reminiscent of the old time emphasis on purgatives and high colonic irrigations of the early 1900s.

Some of the books are expensive and some of the menus advised are difficult and even expensive to follow. Often the reasons for "success" may have a basis in physiological fact but most often the fact is minimized and myth and mystique such as ridding the body of poisons and the magic combinations of food is dominant. Note: Early weight loss is either a result of diuresis or a decrease in energy consumed (total kilocalories for different foods or smaller servings) or energy used (exercise) or all of these.

Three popular weight loss programs are briefly reviewed below:

Weight Watchers — a large national chain of weight control groups (low cost) with some well-developed materials. "Weight Watcher" foods, another company, are very useful for people with diabetes because of labeling. Some local groups may not have nutritive advice of the highest quality. A meeting magazine is available with recipes. Serving sizes need to be stressed. The cost is $12-20 for registration with a weekly fee of $8.[3]

O.A. (Overeaters Anonymous) — Patterned on the alcoholics anonymous regimen. The dietary advice may be poor for people with diabetes, the appetite control and learning to enjoy life with fewer food centered activities may be helpful. O.A. groups are often available every night which help reinforce goal setting. People with diabetes should *not* use the dietary counselling from O.A. personnel. There is no cost nor are special foods involved.[3]

TOPS (Take Off Pounds Sensibly) — A low cost weight control group with much group instruction and control. Some patients find the public criticism unbearable — others find it helpful. The dietary advice often from local people whose only training is successful weight loss may be suspect for people with diabetes. This is a low cost program, $0.25-0.50/week.[3]

Patients with diabetes mellitus should have all dietary plans and materials reviewed by registered dietitians who understand the problems of the disease state. If the menus recommended are appropriate, patients may be allowed to follow them because they can feel part of a "new" adventure and can share experiences with their friends. However, they *must* be made aware of the possibly dangerous or faulty advice that may be given by over-zealous or poorly informed local leaders or group members.

REFERENCES

1. The DCCT Research Groups weight gain associated with intensive therapy in the diabetes control and implications diet: *Diabetes Care*, 11:7:567, July/August 1988.

2. Timely Statement of the American Dietetic Association: Very low calorie weight loss diets. *J Amer Diet Assoc* 89:7: 975, July 1989.

3. Anderson, N., Blum, A.: Crying the Weight Loss Blues, *Changing Times*, April 1989, 75-78.

Section VI:
Dietary Guidelines and Information on Glycemic Index, Dietary Fiber, Sweeteners, and Nutrient Content of Foods

INTRODUCTION

Although nutritional guidelines have been used and described in Sections I and II, some specific published guidelines are described and evaluated in this section. The current Recommended Dietary Allowances[1] are reviewed. The U.S.D.A. Dietary Guidelines, the Food Group Plans (see Glossary) and the American Diabetes Association Energy Distribution Recommendations are included in this section and comments made concerning the value of these for people with diabetes.

SECTION VI: CHAPTER I
NUTRITIONAL GUIDELINES

General Description

As stated earlier in several places, the usual advice in determining diets in the treatment of diabetes is first that these diets should be nutritionally adequate. Although this is a worthy goal, the *first* goal of treatment is control of the disease. The obese person with diabetes probably has stores even of water soluble nutrients and the energy restricted diets by their nature alone encourage nutrient dense foods.

The Recommended Dietary Allowances (RDAs)[1] described here and in other chapters are the NRC-RDAs (see Glossary). The US

RDAs are even higher and were developed for nutrient labeling. The NRC RDAs were developed to apportion food for groups of healthy people. They assume that the nutrients come from *ordinary foods*. This is very important because the nutrients, given in the charts, are representative of all nutrients in the foods. Breakfast foods that are in reality nothing but some grain flakes and a vitamin pill are not appropriate sources of nutrients because the other expected nutrients are not there. Obtaining all of the RDAs for vitamins and minerals from one serving of a food is inappropriate and may mean vitamins and minerals not naturally occurring in foods are added.

Most nutritional evaluations are based on the RDAs and adequacy is sometimes considered 66% of RDAs. There is no scientific basis for this except that the RDA is considered to be an upper limit. The RDAs have usually been revised every five years and often on the basis of expected need rather than research concerning the health of people.

Nutritional adequacy can only be estimated by analysis of food intake using charts. Even laboratory tests are not helpful in terms of stores and therefore long-term adequacy.

Caution:

1. The nutrients for which the RDAs have been established (as well as those for which there are safe levels) are considered to be *representative* or *leader nutrients*. Other nutrients are also present in ordinary foods; not included are supplements added to foods such as in some cereals or sugar based drink mixes.
2. There is no evidence that massive doses of nutrients are protective. Some nutrients are stored and such storage can achieve toxic levels (vitamins A and D are the most common).
3. Nutrient supplements may give a false sense of security and are an expensive "do something" habit. Potential harm can occur from deficiency of "minor" nutrients.
4. There is no way to balance meals nutritionally. Nutritional balance must involve long term intake, consideration of stores and unusual needs, and adequacy of digestion and absorption.

SECTION VI: CHAPTER II
DIETARY GUIDELINES

The Dietary Guidelines were the outcome of the "Dietary Goals" by the Senate Select Committee on Nutrition and Human Needs. They were published with the U.S.D.A. and titled "Nutrition and Your Health, Dietary Guidelines for Americans" in 1980. These guidelines are broad suggestions rather than being specific in amounts and kinds of food. One of the underlying premises of the dietary goals was the prevention of disease.[2] They generally apply to adults.

Dietary Guidelines with Comments for People with Diabetes Mellitus

1. "Eat a variety of foods." This is a worthwhile goal met by the usual diet eaten by people with diabetes. However, the normalization of blood glucose should be approached before radical changes in eating patterns are advised even to meet this goal. If fewer foods are used, identification of "trouble" foods by glucose self-monitoring is easier.

2. "Maintain desirable weight." The goal of achieving and maintaining desirable weight is one of the major goals for treatment of diabetes. However, desirable weight cannot be determined by looking at a table, and a weight loss of 10 to 20 pounds may normalize blood glucose levels for overweight NIDDM people.

3. "Avoid too much fat, saturated fat and cholesterol." Energy controlled diets are normally low in fat which would automatically decrease the intake of saturated fats and cholesterol. Rigid restriction of cholesterol should only be undertaken when physiologically warranted. Low cholesterol diets may be inadvisable for the very young child, the ill and the aged.

4. "Eat foods with adequate starch and fiber." People with diabetes are encouraged to eat foods with complex carbohydrates and unless contraindicated, adequate amounts of fiber.

5. "Avoid too much sugar." Even with liberalization in use of sugar (table sugar) for people with diabetes, the total amount allowed must be a small proportion of the total food intake, except with liquid diets.

6. "Avoid too much sodium." There appears to be no harm in mild restriction of sodium intake and some may benefit from it. Young active people, athletes and active adults should not severely restrict sodium. The palatability of low caloric foods is enhanced with some added salt and if there are no contraindications, the addition of some salt may improve adherence to the diet.

7. "If you drink alcoholic beverages, do so in moderation." The use of alcohol should be carefully evaluated in terms of amounts, kinds and current medications. Alcohol, if used, should always be taken with food, and the energy contribution considered.[3] The metabolism of alcohol does not require insulin, but it contributes a considerable amount of energy (7 kcal/gm or 83 kcal/oz of 100 proof).[4] Alcoholic beverages such as beer, wine and mixed drinks will contribute carbohydrates in varying amounts.

The recommended distribution of energy nutrients by the American Diabetes Association for persons with diabetes are similar to those of the American Heart Association, the National Cancer Institute, the Nutritional Committee for Recommendations for Children with Diabetes of the American Academy of Pediatrics, and the Surgeon General's Report of the Dietary Guidelines for Americans.[3,5] The following are the recommended daily intakes for persons with diabetes—adjustments to be made according to individual need.

Recommended Daily Intakes for Persons with Diabetes Mellitus

1. Carbohydrates: 60% or less of the total energy from carbohydrates. The usual recommendation of 55-60% of the energy as carbohydrates may not be desirable for patients with NIDDM[6] and may present problems for people with high energy needs. The high carbohydrate recommendation encourages the use of sugar which may be contraindicated.

2. Protein: 15-20%. The 0.8 gm/kg body weight[1,5] is probably a better standard for people with either very low or very high intakes of food. Renal patients or potential renal patients may need less protein, whereas pregnant women may need more.

3. Fat: 30% of total energy as fat. This 30% is subdivided into 6-8% polyunsaturated, less than 10% as saturated fat and the remain-

der as monounsaturated fats. One difficulty in applying this recommendation is that foods contain combinations of poly-monounsaturated and saturated fatty acids, and it is impossible to determine the amounts of each type eaten without using food composition tables. Diets low in total energy are usually low in fats. This restriction of total fats rather than emphasis on types may be the best advice in the long run for people with diabetes. People diagnosed as having a type of hyperlipoproteinemia may require individualized instruction.

4. Cholesterol: 300 mg or less per day. Dietary cholesterol may influence blood cholesterol levels but a decrease in total dietary fat may be a more realistic approach. See Section II for cholesterol for children and pregnant women.

5. Fiber: 40 gms or 25 gm/1000 kcal. Current evidence suggests that it may be advisable to increase consumption of whole grains, vegetables and legumes;[5] however, consideration must be given to other nutrients whose availability may be decreased with too much dietary fiber.

SECTION VI: CHAPTER III
FOUR FOOD GROUPS

For many years, attempts have been made to determine food patterns which will provide adequacy (see nutrient needs, Glossary). The most commonly used is the Four Food Groups Guide usually called the Basic Four.[7] Since the "or more" suggestions on each serving size and number has been removed the pattern is now a better one for use in weight control and diabetes than previously. The suggestion that all foods ingested must be from these groups is misleading for people with higher energy needs. Allowances for fats and sugars, except those in fruit, milk, or vetetables, are not made, and the contribution of "other" foods such as desserts, is not considered. Few people who use and advocate the Basic Four actually consider the number and size of servings carefully. One misuse of the guide is to make "so called" balanced meals by including one serving from each group at each meal. This is not appropriate.

The Four Food Group Guide without additional fat in preparation and low fat milk is approximately 1000 kcal and probably marginally adequate for adults. It is difficult to follow the Four Food Group Guide and not meet most of the Recommended Dietary Allowances (the base upon which the plan was made). It is possible to meet the RDAs on other plans. Table 27 lists foods in the Basic Four Group Guide adapted for use with people with diabetes.

SECTION VI: CHAPTER IV
GLYCEMIC EFFECT OF FOODS

Much attention is currently being paid to the glycemic effects of different foods. Some basic information on this is useful.

Glycemic Index

The term, *glycemic index*, has been given to the extent of glycemic response of some carbohydrates in comparison to a standard. Research in this area is useful because it shows graphically that all polysaccharides are not alike in their rate of physiological response. A high glycemic index is not an indication of more energy (kcals) but the rapidity and height of blood glucose elevation in response to a given food in comparison to a standard. Originally the standard was a measured amount of glucose, but currently some researchers[8] are using white bread as the standard. There is still much controversy regarding fiber and glycemic response. Possibly fiber in the diet may impact on glycemic response by delaying gastric emptying time (slow rate of food moving from stomach to small intestine), thus making sugars unavailable for absorption, and/or slowing rate of absorption from the small intestine.

The presence of other food components, i.e., fat and fiber, and the form of the molecule are still being evaluated, as is the food preparation method. Unless the food is taken alone or forms an extremely high proportion of the meal, the glycemic index in an ordinary diet appears to be of relatively little importance except perhaps for ranking starchy foods.[8]

TABLE 27. Basic Four Food Group Guide Adapted for People with Diabetes

Food Groups	Number and Size of Serving	Foods Useful for People with Diabetes	Principal Nutrients in the the Group Foods
Breads and Cereals	4 Servings 1 slice bread or 1/2-3/4 c cereal	All whole grain and enriched flours and products with limited fat	Carbohydrates, proteins, niacin, iron, thiamin, zinc in whole grains, fiber
Fruits and Vegetables	4 Servings 1/3-1/2 c	Lower caloric fruits and vegetables prepared and served without added dressings or sauces	Carbohydrates, small amounts of proteins, vitamin A, C, folacin. Amounts vary with variety
Milk and milk products (does not include butter, cream, cream cheese or margarine)	2 c	Low fat milks, buttermilk, yogurt, cottage cheese and low fat cheeses	Proteins, calcium, riboflavin, zinc, phosphorus, vitamins A, D, B_{12}, lactose in milks, fats in some. milk and cheeses
Meats	Two 2 oz servings of meat	Low fat beef, pork, lamb, fish, poultry, eggs	Proteins, fats iron, zinc, niacin, riboflavin, thiamin, B^6, B^{12}
Beans, lentils, legumes, and nuts vary in protein, carbohydrate and fats and need to be individually calculated.			

Glycemic Effect of Proteins

Amino acid molecules contribute to the energy pool. Excess amino acids are broken into a glucose fraction and a nitrogen containing fraction. The nitrogen is excreted, but the former contribute to the blood glucose level. The amino acids become available for conversion to glucose when the total amount is greater than physiological needs or the needed components of proteins are not available (a lack of appropriate essential amino acids). The estimated amount of protein by weight influencing insulin may be up to 50%. The energy contribution of protein is estimated to be 4 kcal/gm or 120 kcal/oz.

Glycemic Effect of Fat

Fats, whether ingested or stored, have a lesser need for insulin because only 10% of the fat molecule is converted to glucose. Therefore, fats have only a small direct glycemic effect. However, fats present in the digestive tract do tend to slow the rate at which other nutrients are absorbed and may therefore have a significant glycemic effect over a longer period of time. The energy contribution from fats is higher than the other energy nutrients (9 kcal/gm or 255 kcal/oz).

Glycemic Effect of Carbohydrates

In order for carbohydrates to be used by the cells for energy, ingested carbohydrates must be digested, absorbed, circulated in the portal system and made available to the cells by the presence of utilizable insulin. Only limited carbohydrate stores are available in the form of glycogen (stored glucose) in the liver and muscle.

Carbohydrates are classified according to their composition. These classifications are described in the glossary. The energy contribution of carbohydrates is estimated to be 4 kcal/gm or 120 kcal/oz (the same as protein).

SECTION VI: CHAPTER V
SWEETENERS

The refined sugars such as the table sugar (sucrose) have historically been restricted in diabetic diets,[9] but fruits with a high sugar (sucrose, glucose or fructose) content have been allowed. This may be attributed to the use of the term "sugar" (in the blood) to describe diabetes mellitus. Patients frequently refer to their own condition as "I have sugar."

Patients need to understand that sugar as eaten undergoes metabolic changes and that the glucose in the blood is not the identical molecule they have eaten. They also need to understand that sugar in the sugar bowl (sucrose) is the same sucrose that occurs naturally in fruits. Fruits also have other sugars (glucose and fructose).

The chemical classification of sugars is given in the glossary.

The mixture of sugars in fruits is variable. A few examples are given in Table 28. It can be noted that a medium orange contains a little more than one teaspoon of sucrose along with glucose and fructose which makes a total contribution of almost 12 gms of sugars.

As can be seen in the table when fruit or fruit juices are used in recipes as sweeteners (sugar substitutes), one of the principal sweeteners is actually sucrose.

Alternate Sweeteners

Labels of many food products indicate the absence of sugar in the product. However, the list of ingredients may include a variety of sweeteners that can provide the same caloric value as sucrose (see Glossary).

Sugar Alcohols

Sugar alcohols are common in "diatetic" food products. Sorbitol is most often used with mannitol next. Xylitol, although widely used in other countries, is just now being actively marketed in the U.S.[10] The sugar alcohols contain 4 kcal/gm as does sucrose but are not as sweet as sucrose so more has to be used to give the desired sweetness. In addition, products using the sugar alcohols need added fat to give the desired texture. The extra amount of sugar alcohols for sweetness and extra fats for texture can add considerable energy value (kcal) to the food.[11]

Fructose

Fructose is the sweetest of the sugars, and when used by itself, this sweetness is apparent and a smaller amount is used thus reducing the caloric intake slightly. However, in baked products the extra sweetness of fructose is not as apparent and more may be used increasing the caloric value slightly.[12]

Corn syrups are made from corn starch. These contain glucose and fructose but also maltose. Maltose is not as sweet as the two

TABLE 28. Sugar Content of Four Fruits

	Glucose gm	Fructose gm	Sucrose gm	Total Sugar gm
Apple (140 gm) 1 med 3 1/4" dia.	3.2	10.5	4.6	18.4
Peach (87 gm) 1 med	1.0	1.1	4.9	7.6
Banana (114 gm) 1 med	4.8	3.1	7.4	17.8
Orange, navel (140 gm) 2 5/8 " dia.	2.9	3.3	5.5	11.7

Note: Sugar, white, granulated 4 gm (1 tsp) = 3.9 gm sucrose

Source: Matthews, R.H., Pehrsson, P.R., Farhat-Sabet, M.: Sugar Content of Selected Foods: Individual and total sugars. USDA, Human Nutrition Information Services, Home Economics Research Report No. 48, 1987.

simple sugars. The food industry has produced a high fructose corn syrup with about 42-55% of the sugars as fructose. Some manufacturers are now making a highly refined high fructose corn syrup containing 90% fructose which is available as a table top sweetener. Patients are cautioned against using the 42-55% high fructose syrups because they contain 30% or more glucose[13] in addition to the fructose. The highly refined syrups with 90% fructose have not been tested in diabetics.

Honey, molasses and maple syrup are individually described in the glossary. All contain glucose in various amounts and should be treated as table sugars for diabetic patients.

Synthetically Produced Non-Nutritive and Nutritive Sweeteners

Although fats probably are a far greater "threat" to the general public than sugar, the use of sweeteners with few or no calories is growing constantly even for people with diabetes. Fear abounds concerning the safety of "artificial" or non-nutritive sweeteners. No ill effects have been documented in people with diabetes even with years of use. As with any food or food ingredient, excesses should be avoided, especially in the young and pregnant, as a precautionary measure. Below are listed some non-nutritive sweeteners and characteristics of each (also see Glossary).

Cyclamates have been banned in the U.S. since 1970, however, reapproval is expected. It is non-nutritive, 30 times sweeter than sugar, has little or no aftertaste, and can be used in cooking. Other sweeteners are being developed with similar characteristics.

Saccharin is available in tablets and liquids which have no carbohydrates or calories. It has an aftertaste which some find unpleasant. The buffered forms (powders) are packaged with a glucose (dextrose) buffer or lactose or dextrins. Kilocalories from these buffers run from 1-1/2 per packet to 3-1/2. Saccharin use by pregnant women is not recommended. All people, especially young children should exercise moderation in its use.[14]

Aspartame has a brand name of Equal® for powder and of Nutrasweet® in foods. It furnishes 4 kcal per packet (aspartame is made from two amino acids and therefore is actually a nutritive sweetener). It is contraindicated in children with phenylketonuria and people using dopaminergic drugs. Aspartame gives a pleasant taste but disintegrates upon prolonged heating. To date no research has indicated that aspartame use is not safe at ordinary levels of use.[15]

Acesulfame-K (Sunette®) is derived from acetoacetic acid and marketed as Sweet One.™ It contains dextrose and cream of tartar in addition to acesulfame-K. It, like aspartame, is sold in packets which are equivalent in sweetening to 2 tsp of sucrose and contain 4 kcal so it is a nutritive sweetener. Acesulfame-K is heat and pH stable and can be substituted for up to one half of the sugar in baked products.

SECTION VI: CHAPTER VI
DIETARY FIBERS

Introduction

Current research suggests that benefits of increased dietary fiber are more evident when high carbohydrate, low fat diets composed of common foods are used.[16] Concerns about increased fiber intakes for patients with diabetes are related to gastrointestinal problems and possible mineral deficiencies.[14]

Food fibers are commonly classified as soluble (gums, pectins, mucilages) and water insoluble (cellulose, hemicellulose and the non-carbohydrate lignin) (see Glossary). Soluble fibers appear to have the most effect on blood glucose and lipid levels, whereas the insoluble type increase transit time in the gut and aid in relieving constipation and diverticulosis. Caution must be exercised in increasing fiber for the old, inactive patient with limited fluid intakes.

Dietary fiber cannot be considered as a group of distinct components in which one gram of pectin might be compared with one gram of cellulose. Instead, dietary fiber is a complex within each food that will vary not only within the species (growing season, age, etc.) but will also exhibit different characteristics from similar dietary fiber in other foods. In addition, the different materials within the fiber component of a food may have physiological effects which are competing or opposing, or the fibers may have an enhancing effect upon each other.

There is indication that fiber in the food itself is more effective than supplementation of isolated fibers.[16] The current popularity of oat bran appears to be from its high content of mucilages.

The adherence to high fiber diets varies greatly among people with diabetes and appears to be related to dietary changes in general.[17] Some high fiber menus are given in Appendix IX.

The disadvantages of increased intestinal gas, abdominal discomfort, gastrointestinal distress and the altered (decreased) availability of minerals[14] with a high fiber diet must be carefully considered in diets for small children, pregnant women and the elderly.

The addition of fiber to the diet may be contraindicated in persons with diabetes who have gastroporesis. Gastroporesis is thought to occur in 20-30% of persons with diabetes. It develops slowly, decreasing motility and can result in the formation of a bezoar (a compact mass of fibers, skin or other parts of plants and food particles that collect in the stomach or small intestine). Susceptible patients should be counseled to avoid foods with a high fiber content.[18]

Nutrient Contributions of Common Foods

Nutrient contribution is difficult to estimate due to the great variation in food composition, recipes, and serving sizes. The exchange lists are an attempt to simplify these analyses but many difficulties arise. Large numbers of foods have been listed in governmental documents (such as Handbooks 8 and 456, House and Garden Bulletins, etc.) and in privately published books such as Pennington and Church. These are a compilation of data from many sources and are useful estimates of food composition but often do not represent the food a patient actually eats. The analyses of brand-named foods has improved these lists and a more accurate method may be to analyze the recipe rather than by using the food by name. Analyzing a recipe is relatively easy with a computer program.

The large number of computer software programs use data from the government base and food manufacturers' product analyses. A great deal of judgement is necessary to use these programs besides determining serving sizes. The computer evaluation of the diet may use an inappropriate standard for the patient, may be the result of faulty or incomplete data, and may frighten or threaten the patient more than necessary. Computer analysis program results should rarely be given to the patient and never mailed or used without competent dietetic advice.

Even the use of food analysis tables may be misleading. Foods, although made from the same recipe or cooked in the same way, are rarely uniform in nutrient composition. Changes in water content can make significant changes in nutrient contribution when the analysis is determined by weight or measure. Water evaporates rapidly and even breads and pastries will dry out. The computerized food analysis programs give an impression of accuracy that is not deserved because the basis of the data is common with the published one; some items need to be adjusted for the preparation method; and the computer analysis programs generate vast amounts of data which needs to be interpreted by a trained professional knowledgeable in nutrition and data entry. The computer analysis reports give an appearance of accuracy but in fact may not be true. (See Section I for food intake records.)

The often deplored loss of vitamins and minerals from cooking and processing may or may not be significant and is not easily determined. Since the person with diabetes usually has a "better than average" diet, food preparation and storage loss of the vitamins and minerals (most noticeable in terms of ascorbic acid, thiamin and folacin) will not be detailed. Instead, the caution is made to view food analysis by chart carefully and recommend a variety of foods.

The energy which is available from food is measured in the United States in kilocalories (kcal) (see Glossary). Although kilocalories and megaJoules (mJ) are both used in Great Britain, the use of megaJoules is more common in many European countries (see Glossary).

The amount of energy available in the body from one gram of carbohydrate is assumed to be 4 kilocalories in the U.S. The amount of carbohydrate in foods listed in charts is often found by subtracting the energy from protein and fats from the total energy and the remainder is considered from carbohydrate.[19] There is evidence that carbohydrates contribute different amounts of energy according to the saccharide category with polysaccharides furnishing more energy per unit of weight than mono- or disaccharides because of the fewer water molecules in the structure.

No research has been found by the authors on differences in efficiency of absorption in people of different ages or with diabetes. It is possible the obese person has very efficient absorption and conversion of energy. If this were found to be true, then, for example, if a person actually obtained 4.1 kcal from each gram of carbohydrate instead of 4 kcal/gm, this could account for as much as four pounds in one year more than estimated.

Some representative foods and their caloric contribution are listed in Appendix XI.

REFERENCES

1. Food and Nutrition Board, National Research Council: *Recommended Dietary Allowances*, 10th revised ed.: Washington, D.C., National Academy of Sciences, 1989.

2. Cronin, F.J., Shaw, A.M.: Summary of dietary recommendations for healthy Americans. *Nutr. Today* 23:6:26, Nov/Dec 1988.

3. American Diabetic Association Position Statement: Nutritional recommendations and principles of individuals with diabetes mellitus. *Diabetes Care* 10:1:126, Jan/Feb 1987.

4. Pennington, J.A.T.: *Bowes and Church's Food Values of Portions Commonly Used*. 15th ed: Philadelphia: Lippencott, 1989.

5. U.S. Dept of Health and Human Services: *The Surgeon General's Report on Nutrition and Health*. U.S. DHHS Publ No. 88-50211. Washington, D.C. 1988.

6. Hollenbeck, C., Coulston, A.M., Reaven, G.M.: Effects of sucrose on carbohydrate and lipid metabolism on NIDDM patients, *Diabetes Care* 12:1:62, Jan 1989.

7. Haughton, V., Gussow, J.D., Dodds, J.M.: An historical study of the underlying assumptions for United States Food Guides from 1917 through the Basic Four Food Groups Guide. *J Nutr Ed* 19:4:169, Jul/Aug 1987.

8. Jenkins, D.J.A., Wolever, T.M.S., Jenkins, A.L.: Starchy foods and glycemic index. *Diabetes Care* 11:2:149, Feb 1988.

9. American Diabetes Association Task Force, Crapo, P.A. Chrm. Nutritional recommendations and principles for individuals with diabetes mellitus: 1986. *Diabetes Care* 10:1:126, Jan/Feb 1987.

10. Voster, M.: Letter and comments: Xylitol. *Diabetes Care* 12:2:171, Feb 1989.

11. Crapo, P. and Powers, M.A.: Alias: Sugar. *Diabetes Forecast* pg 22, Mar/Apr 1981.

12. ADA Reports: Position of the American Dietetic Association: Appropriate use of nutritive and non-nutritive sweeteners, *J. Am Diet Assoc*, 87:12:1689, 1987.

13. Crapo, P.A., Olefsky, J.M.: Fructose — its characteristics, physiology, and metabolism. *Nutr Today*, 15:4:10, Jul/Aug 1980.

14. Anderson, J.W.: Nutrition management of diabetes mellitus. Chapt 57 in *Modern Nutrition in Health and Disease* 7th ed. Edited by Shils, M.E. and Young, V.R.: Philadelphia Lea and Febiger 1988.

15. Filer, L.J. and Stenzink, L.O.: Aspartame metabolism in normal adults, phenylketonuric heterozygotes and diabetic subjects. *Diabetes Care* 12:1 Supplement 1:67, Jan 1989.

16. Vinik, A. and Jenkins, D.J.A.: Dietary fiber in management of diabetes. *Diabetes Care* 11:2:160, Feb 1988.

17. Kouris A., Wahlquist, M.L., and Worsley, A.: Characteristics that enhance adherence to high-carbohydrate/high-fiber diets by persons with diabetes. *J Am Diet Assoc* 88:11:1422, Nov 1988.

18. Emerson, A.P.: Foods high in fiber and phytobezoar formation. *J Am Diet Assoc* 87:12:1675, Dec 1987.

19. Watt, B.K. and Merrill, A.L.: Composition of foods — Raw, Processed, Prepared. *U.S. Dept. of Agr. Handbook* 8(rev) 1963.

APPENDIXES

List of Appendixes

Page

Appendix I

Height/Weight Tables
Estimating Body Weight (Adults)
Median Heights and Weights
and Recommended Energy Intake (RDA)

Height-Weight Tables
Estimating Body Weight (Adults)

Several different height-weight charts exist (see Glossary). Most are based on the assumption that low weight per height is best, although many healthy people may weigh less or more than the figures given.

Formulas for estimating body weight also exist. Probably the best known one is the easy method given below. Since "ideal" body weight is unknown and body weight has to be calculated at times for transcribing diets some reference body weight has to be chosen as "acceptable" for these purposes. Height-weight tables are included here and one method of estimation of body weight given.

1. Estimation of body weight (adults)
2. Metropolitan Life Insurance Table of Height-Weight

1.   BODY WEIGHT BY ESTIMATION (ADULTS)

Build	Women	Men
Medium	Allow 100 lb for the first 5 ft of height, plus 5 lb for each additional inch.	Allow 106 lb for the first 5 ft of height, plus 6 lb for each additional inch.
Small	Subtract 10%	Subtract 10%
Large	Add 10%	Add 10%

Ref.: Hamwi, G.J.: Therapy: Changing Dietary Concepts. Chapter XVII in Diabetes Mellitus: Diagnosis and Treatment, Vol I. Danowski, T.S. Ed., New York, American Diabetes Assoc, 1964, p 74.

2. HEIGHT-WEIGHT TABLES

New height-weight tables based on insurance records have been published by the Metropolitan Life Insurance Co. of New York. It is the standard used by virtually everyone in the insurance industry and health professions. The company first devised these tables in 1943, revised them in 1959, but did no further alterations until the 1983 tables. Differences between the 1959 and 1983 tables appear to be due to changes in lifestyle. The weight ranges should not be construed as "ideal".

Height and Weight Table

WOMEN[1]

Height Ft In	Small Frame	Medium Frame	Large Frame
4 10	102-111	109-121	118-131
4 11	103-113	111-123	120-134
5 0	104-115	113-126	122-137
5 1	106-118	115-129	125-140
5 2	108-121	118-132	128-143
5 3	111-124	121-135	131-147
5 4	114-127	124-138	134-151
5 5	117-130	127-141	137-155
5 6	120-133	130-144	140-159
5 7	123-136	133-147	143-163
5 8	126-139	136-150	146-167
5 9	129-142	139-153	149-170
5 10	132-145	142-156	152-173
5 11	135-148	145-159	155-176
6 0	138-151	148-162	158-179

According to source, weights at ages 25-59 based on lowest mortality. Weight in pounds according to frame (in indoor clothing weighing three pounds, shoes with one-inch heels).

[1] Source: Metropolitan Life Insurance Company, 1983 Height and Weight Tables

Height and Weight Table

MEN[1]

Height Ft In	Small Frame	Medium Frame	Large Frame
5 2	128–134	131–141	138–150
5 3	130–136	133–143	140–153
5 4	132–138	135–145	142–156
5 5	134–140	137–148	144–160
5 6	136–142	139–151	146–164
5 7	138–145	142–154	149–168
5 8	140–148	145–157	152–172
5 9	142–151	148–160	155–176
5 10	144–154	151–163	158–180
5 11	146–157	154–166	161–184
6 0	149–160	157–170	164–188
6 1	152–164	160–174	168–192
6 2	155–168	164–178	172–197
6 3	158–172	167–182	176–202
6 4	162–176	171–187	181–207

According to source, weights at ages 25–59 based on lowest mortality. Weight in pounds according to frame (in indoor clothing weighing five pounds, shoes with one-inch heels).

[1] Source: Metropolitan Life Insurance Company, 1983 Height and Weight Tables.

Median Heights and Weights and Recommended Energy Intake

Category	Age (years)	Weight (kg)	Weight (lb)	Height (cm)	Height (in)	Average Energy Allowance (kcal) Per kg	Per lb	Per day
Infants	0.0-0.5	6	13	60	24	108	49	650
	0.5-1.0	9	20	71	28	98	45	850
Children	1 – 3	13	29	90	35	102	46	1300
	4 – 6	20	44	112	44	90	41	1800
	7 – 10	28	62	132	52	70	32	2000
Males	11 – 14	45	99	157	62	55	25	2500
	15 – 18	66	145	176	69	45	20	3000
	19 – 24	72	160	177	70	40	18	2900
	25 – 50	79	174	176	70	37	17	2900
	51 +	77	170	173	68	30	14	2300
Females	11 – 14	46	101	157	62	47	21	2200
	15 – 18	55	120	163	64	40	18	2200
	19 – 24	58	128	164	65	38	17	2200
	25 – 50	63	138	163	64	36	16	2200
	51 +	65	143	160	63	30	14	1900
Pregnancy								+300
Lactation								+500

Source: Recommended Dietary Allowances, 10th ed.: Washington, D.C., National Academy of Sciences, 1989.

The heights and weights of the reference adults are the actual medians for the U.S. population of the specific ages taken from HANES II Study. These figures should not be considered as "ideal" or "desirable" The medians for ages under 19 were adapted for the RDAs from the work of Hamill, et al.

Reference: Hamill, P.V.V., Drizd, T.A., Johnson, C.L., Reed, R.B., Roche, A.F. and Moore, W.M., 1979. Physical Growth: National Center for Health Statistics Percentiles. Am J Clin Nutr 32:607, 1979.

The energy allowances for adults are for men and women engaged in light to moderate activity. The allowances for older age represents mean energy needs over this age span allowing for a 2 to 3 percent decrease in resting metabolic rate per decade and a reduction in activity after age 51 of 600 kcal/day for men and of 300 kcal/day for women. Energy allowances for children under age 10 were estimated from energy intakes of children these ages associated with normal growth.

Appendix II

Estimation of Energy Needs

Estimation of Energy Needs

Clinical methods are available for determining energy use. These are based on oxygen utilization and carbon dioxide production. Caution is advised in use of charts especially the popular ones of the number of minutes to use a certain number of calories. These sometimes include energy for basal functions and usually disregard surface area, muscle mass, training, age, sex, and aftereffect of exercise.

Included in this section are:

1. Formula for calculating basal energy used.
2. Estimating total energy expenditure (in kcal) for basic functions and activity.

1. Calculation for Basal Energy Used:

Harris Benedict Method for estimating basal energy expenditure (BEE).

Men: BEE = $66.5 + (13.8 \times W) + (5 \times H) - (6.8 \times A)$

Women: BEE = $65.5 + (9.6 \times W) + (1.8 \times H) - (4.7 \times A)$

W = weight in kilograms
H = height in centimeters
A = age in years

Adaptation of Harris Benedict for Total Energy Use[1]. Add

20% of BEE for Sedentary
35% of BEE for Moderately active
50% of BEE for Active

Add for fever or stress
13% of BEE for one degree
centigrade for fever, 10-100%
of BEE for surgery, fracture,
or burns.

[1] Source of these figures is obscure and
varies slightly in different references.

2. Estimating Total Energy Use (in kcal) for
   Basic Functions and Activity.

The lowest level of energy expenditure
is when the body is sleeping or lying
quietly. These body functions are termed
basal or resting metabolism depending upon
the conditions under which the measurements
of oxygen utilization and carbon dioxide
production are taken.

During the sleeping-resting periods the
body tissues require energy for their
functions, but all tissues do not need the
same amounts. The brain which accounts for
only about 2.3% of body weight utilizes
about the same amount of energy as do the
skeletal muscles which can account for up to
50% of body weight. The metabolism of
adipose tissue at rest is similar to the
resting utilization of brain and muscle.

The energy expenditure of the brain and
adipose tissue remains almost constant
throughout the day. However, muscle tissue
when used during exercise can increase its
energy expenditure as much as a hundred
times the amount of energy expended by
resting muscles.

The ability of muscle tissue to utilize large amounts of energy for activity is the basis for classification of activities by levels of intensity, i.e. relative energy expenditures.

Some general guidelines for assessing the energy expenditure of activities are listed below:

1. The number and size of muscles used. Sitting requires the expenditure of only a small amount of energy beyond that required while lying down sleeping or resting. Small hand and arm movements while sitting require only a small additional energy expenditure over that required for resting metabolism.

When the large muscles, especially in the legs, move the entire body the energy expenditure increases. The larger the body being moved, the greater the energy used.

2. The speed of the muscle activity also increases the energy expended particularly when the larger muscles are involved. There can be a sizeable increase in energy expended as the pace of walking becomes faster. Running will expend even more energy.

3. Moving (lifting) the body upwards as when climbing stairs or walking up an incline requires a large amount of energy. The muscles have to work hard to lift the body weight up stairs or up a hill. While this activity has a high energy cost it is seldom of long duration so unless climbing stairs is a major part of a daily occupation, it

would increase daily energy expenditure only slightly.

4. Moving the body down stairs or down an incline also requires more energy expenditure than just walking on level ground because work has to be done to keep the body from falling down. As in the case above, the duration of the descent would have more effect on the energy expended than just the activity itself.

5. Duration of the activity has been referred to above in lifting and lowering the body. Any activity will require more energy the longer it is carried on regardless of the intensity of the activity.

6. Trained muscles require less energy to perform an activity than do untrained ones. When a person starts to do an activity such as tennis, he will use considerably more energy than when he becomes an expert.

7. Moving the body over very rough ground requires more energy than walking on an even surface. Walking in wet sand or mud when the feet have to be pulled up with each step is hard work.

8. Carrying a heavy load (such as a child or groceries) requires more energy. This is the same situation as moving a larger body. The more weight the muscles have to move, the more energy is expended.

9. Climate – Climatic conditions appear to have little effect on energy expenditure except under extreme conditions. In a very cold environment, the weight of extra clothing would increase the energy cost of the activity.

10. Age – A child before 2-3 years expends energy for basal/resting metabolism at a higher rate than at any other time of life. This rate gradually decreases throughout life. By age 85, the rate will be about 85% of the value at age 25.

Some studies have shown that the decreased working capacity with aging may be associated with a reduced ability of the body to supply muscles with sufficient oxygen and nutrients. This would indicate a reduced capacity for energy expenditures in activities.

Ref.: Durnin, J.V.G.A. and Passmore, R.: Energy, Work and Leisure. London. Heinemann Educational Books, Ltd. 1967.

The following materials show:
1. Normal values for energy expenditure (kcal/hour) for resting metabolism in young adults. Values are given for both sexes of various body types and for different weights.
2. Energy expenditure (kcal/hour) in activities of different levels of intensity for a representative young adult female and male. Figures include the energy expended for basal functions and the activity.
3. Form that can be used to record activities.
4. Form for calculating estimated total energy expenditure (kcal).

Normal Values for Energy Expenditure (kcal/hour) for Resting Metabolism in Young Adults

Classification Men	Classification Women	Body Fat (%)	Body Weight kg/lb							
			45 100	50 110	55 120	60 132	65 143	70 154	75 165	80 176
Thin		5		60	64	67	71	76	79	83
Average		10		56	61	65	68	73	77	80
Plump	Thin	15	50	53	58	62	65	70	74	78
Fat	Average	20	47	50	55	59	63	67	71	75
	Plump	25		48	52	56	60	64	68	72
	Fat	30			49	53	57	61	65	69

Source: Durnin, J.V.G.A. and Passmore, R.: Energy, Work And Leisure, London. Heinemann Educational Books, Ltd, 1967

Energy Expenditure (kcal) per Hour in Activities of Different Levels of Intensity

Level	Intensity	Activity Classification	Range of kcal/hr – Young Adults* Women 55 kg/ 120 lbs	Men 75 kg/ 165 lbs
0		Sleeping or lying down	55	77
I	Sedentary	Eating, Knitting, Playing cards, Sewing, Sitting quitely, Studying, Typing	60-64	78-114
II	Very Light Activity	Driving car, Ironing, Lab work, Peeling vegetables, Taking care of personal necessities, Sweeping floor	90-114	120-150
III	Light Activity	Cooking, Dishwashing, Doing hand laundry, Golfing (expert), Normal walking, Washing floors with mop	120-134	156-300

Energy Expenditure (cont.)

			240-354	306-450
IV	Moderate Activity	Cleaning vigorously	Playing table tennis	
		Cleaning windows	Playing volley ball	
		Gardening	Walking down Golfing stairs	
		Moving furniture	Rapid walking	
		Making beds	Washing car	
			360+	456+
V	Heavy Activity	Bicycling	Swimming	
		Dancing	Playing tennis	
		Football	Walking up stairs	
		Gymnastics	Running	
		Hard labor		
		Basketball		

Source: Durnin, J.V.G.A. and Passmore, R. Energy, Work and Leisure: London,
Heinemann Educational Books Ltd. 1967

* Energy expenditure for activity levels I-V includes energy cost of metabolic activities.

Activity Record

Name:

Time From To	Time Spent	Activity	Levels					
			0 At Rest or Sleeping	I Seden-tary	II Very Light Exercise	III Light Exercise	IV Moderate Exercise	V Heavy Exercise

150

Form for Calculating Total Energy Expenditure (kcal)

Level of Intensity	Hours	(kcal/hr)	Estimated kcal
Sleeping or Resting	___	___	___
I. Sedentary Activity	___	___	___
II. Very Light Activity	___	___	___
III. Light Activity	___	___	___
IV. Moderate Activity	___	___	___
V. Heavy Activity	___	___	___

Total Estimated Energy Expenditure - 24 hours ___

Appendix III

Forms for Estimating
and Recording Dietary Intake

Food Information Sheet

Name:_____ Phone:_____

Age:____ Height:_____ Present Wt.____ lbs

Recent Loss:_____ Recent Gain:_____

Work (Kind & Hours):_____

School (Name & Hours):_____

Leisure or Sports/Activities:_____

How Often:_____

1. What are your favorite meals/snacks:
Meals
At Home _____

Away from Home _____
Snacks
At Home _____

Away from Home _____

2. At what time (hour) do usually eat?

A.M._____ Noon_____

P.M._____ Evening_____

3. How is your schedule different over
   weekends/holidays? _____
   _____

4. What do you plan to do about your food
   and controlling diabetes? What help do
   you need? _____
   _____

24-Hour Recall Food Intake

Please tell me everything you had to eat
and drink since this time yesterday.

Use probe questions such as:

>At what times did you eat?
>
>At what times did you have anything
>to drink?
>
>What did you eat or drink?
>
>How much?
>
>How was it fixed?
>
>Anything added?
>
>Butter, Margarine?
>
>Oil, Dressing?
>
>Sugar?
>
>Any other snack?
>
>Were your meals yesterday like what
>you eat most days?
>
>How many days a week are different?

24-Hour Dietary Recall Form

Name:_____

Date:_____

In:_____

Counselor:_____

Time	Food	Amount/ Description	Energy/ Nutrient Estimate

Name:_____

Date:_____

Energy Intake for 24 Hours

Time	Food Beverage	Amount/ Description	CHO	PRO	FAT	kcal

Totals

Date: _____

Food Intake Calculation Sheet

Name: _____

Food	Portion (amount)	Energy (kcal)	PRO g	FAT g	CHO g	FIBER g	Ca mg	P mg	Fe mg	Vit A I.U.	Vit B$_1$ mg	Ribo mg	Niac mg	Vit C mg	% Energy PRO CHO FAT

Activity/Food Record

Name: _____   Date: _____

Time From To	No. of Minutes	Activity	Food	Kind	Amount	Comments

159

Inventory to Estimate Saturated Fat and Cholesterol Intake

For each of the following foods choose the answer that represents how often you eat the food. Use the following numbers to find your points.

Frequently Points
Never 0
Eat about once a month 1
Eat about twice a month 2
Eat at least one a week 3
Eat about 3 times a week 4
Eat daily 5

Food	Points
1. Hamburger	_____
2. Hot Dogs	_____
3. Fried Chicken	_____
4. Bacon/Ham	_____
5. Roast Beef	_____
6. Potato Chips/French Fries	_____
7. Doughnuts	_____
8. Croissant/Sweet Rolls	_____
9. Pie/Cake	_____
10. Pizza	_____
11. Regular Milk/Chocolate Milk	_____
12. Low Fat Milk	_____
13. Ice Cream	_____
14. Chocolate Candy Bars	_____
15. "Real" Butter	_____
16. Margarine	_____
17. Salad Dressing (Regular 2-3 tsp)	_____
18. Gravy	_____
19. Snack Crackers	_____
20. Fried Foods	_____
Total Points	_____

Scoring 50 or more -- Intake way too much
40 - 49   -- Intake too high
30 - 39   -- Intake high
20 - 29   -- Intake OK
0 - 19   -- Intake low

Appendix IV

Food Choice Plan
Instruction for Patients

Food Choice Plan

Goals of Food Choice Plan

1. To make achievement of euglycemia and weight control the primary goals of treatment.

2. To shorten the adaptation time, physiologically and psychologically, to food intake management.

3. To provide an individualized program and, therefore, a contract that can allow for special needs, schedules and food preference.

4. To furnish an easy reporting/monitoring system so that questions are answered and changes when needed are made quickly.

5. To streamline the diet history/planning system by having the patient choose familiar foods within the energy prescription.

6. To forbid no foods and to teach serving sizes as the control method of food intake.

7. To postpone detailed systems such as exchange lists until euglycemia is approached.

8. To allow for additional restrictions such as sodium or fats if necessary.

Protocol

1. Physician ascertains patient is able and willing to assume responsibility for planning food intake and makes a referral to the dietitian. The energy (caloric) prescription is necessary.

2. The dietitian gives the patient a worksheet and explains system.

3. Patient writes menus for three days with no restrictions except total energy and any other necessary restrictions actually prescribed by the physician.

4. The dietitian reviews the menus and prescribes serving sizes and appropriate preparation methods. Patient chooses alternate items if desired.

5. Enough copies of Food Choice Plan approved in item 4 are then duplicated for the patient to mail back before the follow-up phone call. Patient is instructed to record all alternate or omitted foods.

6. Phone call by the dietitian at 1-2 weeks, necessary appointments made and additional information given.

7. One month following visit to the dietitian, review Food Choice Plan to accomplish weight loss, changes in schedules, blood glucose values.

8. Monitoring by mail, phone, or office
    visit for three more months.

Key Points of Plan

1. Monitor intake.
2. Review patient records.
3. Check patient's understanding of
    serving sizes and food choices.
4. Provide patient with a list of foods
    with their caloric values early in
    treatment.
5. Keep accurate records of weight
    changes.
6. If success is not achieved search for
    problem foods, stresses or
    misinformation.

Patient Instructions

Here are some suggestions for making the
Food Choice Plan work for you:

Step I.   Your Prescription: Visit your
           physician and receive your
           calorie prescription (this is
           your calorie budget).
           You should receive a sample Plan
           that will be your worksheet.

Step II.   Your Worksheet:
           On your FCP worksheet write a
           foods for Menu I. Your menu
           should include everything you
           plan to eat in one day. List as
           well the times you plan to eat
           and the size of the servings.

           Menu I should be the schedule you
           use most of the time.

Write in exact foods and how much
you plan to eat. Put what kind
of food (example, hamburgers, not
meat, apple, not fruits, etc.)

List how the food is prepared
(example: fried, baked).

Add all items such as butter,
catsup, gravy and so on, and
beverages and snacks.

Step III. <u>Plan Menu II</u>:
If your activities are very much
alike every day, then Menu II
would be much like Menu I but
with different foods.

If some days you eat fewer meals
or exercise more or get up later,
Menu II should be written for
that kind of day.

Step IV. <u>Plan Menu III</u>: This a good place
to plan for parties, travel,
special functions, eating in
restaurants or if necessary when
you don't feel well.

Step V. <u>Worksheet Check</u>: Have your
worksheet checked by your
dietitian. If you have a low
calorie budget you may have to
eat small servings or only eat
one favorite a meal. No food is
forbidden entirely. You may have
some restrictions such as salt or
fat if your physician has ordered
this.

Step VI. <u>Record Form Made</u>: Rewrite your approved Plan. Duplicate enough copies of your approved plan to use until your next visit to the dietitian. Use a different copy of the approved plan each day as a record.

Step VII. <u>Keeping Your Food Record</u>: Date each record. Check all the food on the Food Choice Plan that you actually ate each day. If you ate a different amount than planned or ate different foods, record this under Alternates exactly what changes you made. If you ate one menu exactly as planned, you may just check the whole menu. Be sure to note omitted as well as added foods.

Step VIII. <u>Revision if Necessary</u>: If you are using a large number of alternates or the calorie budget is not working, contact your dietitian to make a new menu plan. Start at Step I again.

Step IX. <u>Month Checkup</u>: Your physician and dietitian will want to check your Food Choice Plan the first time after a month, maybe sooner. Telephone checks are helpful as well.

Step X. <u>Habits Formed</u>: If your food budget works well, you will be able to change menu items as time goes on and become very good at choosing the right amount of each. Keep your plan exactly for one month and very closely for two months, until you and your body have become adjusted to the routine.

Some suggestions if you have a limited food budget. (Low caloric diet.)

1) Watch serving sizes; a glass, spoon or plate may be bigger than you think.
2) Check amount of fruit. It is a good idea to eat only whole fruit, not juice unless juice is important to you.
3) If you have Type II diabetes, don't eat more than three meals a day and have 4-5 hours between meals.
4) Foods with fiber make you feel fuller.
5) Diluting foods such as soup with water makes a serving size seem even bigger.
6) Watch out especially for fats and alcohol. Fats are often used in preparation.
7) Read labels, dietetic foods have calories - often a lot of them.
8) Keep in touch with your medical team.

Food Choice Plan
Use a form for each day

Name: _____   Date: _____

Time	MENU I		MENU II		MENU III		Comments
	Food	Serv. Size	Food	Serv. Size	Food	Serv. Size	

Directions: 1. Check or circle the food you ate.
2. Change time and/or amount if different.
3. Record all alternate or additional foods and amounts.

168

Appendix V

Information Test and Answers
Attitude Survey

Information Test

Name:_____
Date:_____
Date of Diagnosis:_____
Diet Prescription:_____

This test is for people who <u>are</u> taking insulin. In order to answer the questions below, circle:

O   if you don't know.

F   if you are sure the statement is wrong.

PF   if you are not sure but you think it is probably false.

PT   if you are not sure but you think it is probably true.

T   if you are sure it is true.

1. I can eat almost everything if I eat the right amount   O F PF PT T

2. The food I eat makes no difference as long as I don't eat sugar.   O F PF PT T

3. Eating at restaurants is possible.   O F PF PT T

4. Scheduling my food can make a real difference in how I feel.   O F PF PT T

5. I'll have to eat <u>dietetic</u> foods while everyone else eats ordinary foods.   O F PF PT T

6. The foods on my food plan are good for everyone.   O F PF PT T

7. I need to take vitamin pills.   O F PF PT T

8. Before exercising, I should take extra food.   O F PF PT T

9. Alcoholic beverages are allowed for people with diabetes.   O F PF PT T

10. A large (3 inch) raw apple has as much carbohydrate (sugar) as a two ounce chocolate bar.   O F PF PT T

11. Honey affects insulin and has the same calories as sugar.   O F PF PT T

12. Starches such as flour have the same calories as sugar. O F PF PT T

13. I can use as much artificial sweetener as I want.   O F PF PT T

14. Basic nutritive requirements are the same for people whether they have diabetes or not.   O F PF PT T

15. The sugar in fruit affects insulin differently than table sugar.   O F PF PT T

16. A person with diabetes needs to consider proteins and fats as well as carbohydrates.   O F PF PT T

17. People get diabetes because they eat too much sugar.   O F PF PT T

18. Calories in foods are often "hidden".   O F PF PT T

19. Eating fiber will cure my diabetes.   O F PF PT T

20. Cough syrups, laxatives, and other remedies have sugar in them.   O F PF PT T

21. Any source of sugar can be used to treat an insulin reaction.   O F PF PT T

22. Hard "fats" such as those in meats have more effect on insulin than soft fats such as oils.   O F PF PT T

Answers to Information Test

1. I can eat almost everything if
   I eat the right amount.   TRUE

   If you are willing to plan for the foods you are going to eat and watch the serving sizes, almost any food can be calculated in your plan. Learning what foods contain and how each food effects your blood glucose gives you control of your food choices.

2. The food I eat makes no difference as long as I don't eat
   sugar.   PROB FALSE

   Scheduling your food and your insulin are the biggest factors in daily control of your blood glucose. When you eat, the serving sizes you choose and the food composition are all important. Sugar content is only one component of this.

3. Eating at restaurants is possible.
                        TRUE

   Your dietitian can teach you to know what to order so you can stay on your food plan. You need to plan carefully the time you will be served and watch the total amount of food if you eat crackers or something while you are waiting to be served.

4. Scheduling my food can make a real
   difference in how I feel.   TRUE

Planning a schedule that fits your life style is of greatest importance. What to eat, when to eat, how much to eat are factors as well as exercise, sleep and understanding what to do if you have to change your schedule. Knowing how to control these will put you in charge of your schedule.

5. I'll have to eat <u>dietetic</u> foods while everyone else eats ordinary foods.
                                    FALSE

Although <u>dietetic</u> foods do not usually have table sugar (sucrose) in them, they often have other sugars such as sorbitol and xylitol and often extra fat. Dietetic candies and sweets <u>must</u> be calculated in your food plan.

6. The foods on my food plan are good for everyone.   TRUE

Since your food plan is based on a variety of ordinary foods in planned amounts, the foods you eat are the same as everyone else's. You may not be able to eat large servings or have more than one high calorie food at a time, but neither can lots of other people.

7. I need to take vitamin pills.
                                PROB FALSE

If you follow a good food plan you probably will get all the vitamins you need as well as the other nutrients in foods. Vitamin pills <u>do not</u> make up for a poor diet and large amounts may even be harmful.

The main purpose of your food plan is to help control your diabetes. Since you need to follow a food plan for years, your dietitian will help you choose food to meet your nutrient needs.

8. Before exercising, I should take extra food.   TRUE

If you take insulin, you do need to consider if you need extra food while exercising. <u>Do not</u> cut out the insulin and be careful about taking too much food. Blood sugar should be checked before exercising. Planning for regular exercise is important and of course you should have some glucose available.

9. Alcoholic beverages are allowed for people with diabetes.   PROB TRUE

Alcohol does contribute calories and does have an effect on blood sugar. Many alcoholic beverages also contain carbohydrates (sugars) so <u>any</u> alcohol intake should be discussed with your physician. Sometimes people do not follow their diets after they consume alcohol - this is dangerous too.

10. A large (3 inch) raw apple has as much carbohydrate (sugar) as a two ounce chocolate bar.   TRUE

The candy bar has more calories (300 kcal) (the apple has 133 kcal) because it has fat in it, but the big apple has slightly more sugar depending on the size of the apple. The calories in the chocolate bar came from fat, although fat has less effect on blood glucose than carbohydrates and proteins, the calories from fats and the possible effects of a high fat diet need to be considered. The fiber and vitamins in the apple help make it a better choice as well.

11. Honey affects insulin and has the
     same calories as sugar.   TRUE

Honey actually has more sugar per tablespoon than table sugar, and it has about the same effect on insulin and blood sugar. The amount of other nutrients (vitamins and minerals) are so small that honey has no advantage. Both honey and table sugar are partly fructose, even though honey has more fructose, the effect on blood sugar in ordinary amounts is the same.

12. Starches such as flours have the same
     calories as sugar.   PROB TRUE

The body gets approximately the same number of calories from starches in flour, rice and potatoes as it does from sugar. Starches are often advised in place of sugar because most starch foods have vitamins and minerals in them. Much research is now being done concerning the effects of different starches on blood sugar, and the length of time it takes for different starches to get into the blood stream varies. In ordinary amounts as part of meals, these different rates probably have little influence on your blood glucose.

13. I can use as much artificial sweetener
     as I want.   PROB FALSE

Although most people use artificial sweeteners, you can "over dose". Moderation is best.

14. Basic nutritive requirements are the same for people whether they have diabetes of not.   TRUE

People of all ages and conditions need the same nutrients; they may need them in different amounts. The people who choose good varied diets and keep their diabetes under control usually have very nutritious food as well.

15. The sugar in fruits affects insulin differently than table sugar.

PROB FALSE

The sugar in fruit juice is diluted with water and fruit has vitamins and minerals. The sugar in whole fruit will have some fiber with it and that may have some effect. Some of the sugar in fruits is identical to table sugar (sucrose) and the rest is fructose which is also part of sucrose.

16. A person with diabetes needs to consider proteins and fats as well as carbohydrates.   TRUE

Fats contribute the most calories. They also make food taste better and give us a feeling of fullness. Proteins can be used (partly) as a carbohydrate by the body. You need enough and the right kinds of proteins but excess proteins and fats affect your disease.

17. People get diabetes because they eat too much sugar.   FALSE

The term "sugar" diabetes came from the fact that the urine had sugar in it. Eating sugar did not cause the disease. All food components need to be considered by people who take insulin not just sugar.

18. Calories in foods are often "hidden".
                                          TRUE

If a food tastes "rich" and "creamy", it usually has extra fat. Crisp fried foods have extra fat too. Rich and sweet foods may have extra sugar as may tender cakes. Tender meats often have extra fat as well. Your dietitian can help you learn to detect these "hidden" calories.

19. Eating fiber will cure my diabetes.
                                          FALSE

Increasing fiber in the diet has been found to be helpful in controlling diabetes, helping people lose weight, and helping people with constipation. Your food plan should include a good amount of fiber for you.

20. Cough syrups, laxatives and other remedies have sugar in them.
                                          TRUE

Some laxatives such as Metamucil^{TM} are marketed without sugar as well. Read labels carefully.

21. Any source of sugar can be used to treat an insulin reaction.

                                        TRUE

Glucose tablets are the fastest, but the best sugar is the sugar closest at hand -- life savers, sugar packets, honey, soft drinks, etc.

22. Hard "fats" such as those in meats have more effect on insulin than soft fats such as oils.   FALSE

The effect of fats on insulin is little, but the effect of fats on the arteries and veins may be important, so less total fat and use of oils is usually advised. Taking in less total fat helps with weight control too.

Attitude Survey

Name:_____ Date:_____

Please mark your opinion on the following statements:

Circle   (1) if you strongly disagree
           (2) if you disagree at least
               a little
           (3) if it doesn't matter or
               you think it is not
               important (4) if you agree
           somewhat
           (5) if you strongly agree

		SD D N A SA
1.	My diet is the easiest part of my treatment.	1 2 3 4 5
2.	The correct choices of foods are easy to understand.	1 2 3 4 5
3.	As far as food is concerned, I can be like anyone else in the foods I eat.	1 2 3 4 5
4.	With my schedule, I can stick to a diet.	1 2 3 4 5
5.	The regulations about food are easy.	1 2 3 4 5
6.	I don't have to give up any food.	1 2 3 4 5
7.	I can go to parties and eat big meals.	1 2 3 4 5

8. I can eat out in rest-
   aurants.   1 2 3 4 5

9. I don't have to have special
   foods.   1 2 3 4 5

10. Foods I like are in my diet.   1 2 3 4 5

11. I know I can manage the
    diet.   1 2 3 4 5

12. My family and friends will
    learn this diet easily.   1 2 3 4 5

13. The diet is a very important
    part of treatment.   1 2 3 4 5

14. I can change my food habits
    easily.   1 2 3 4 5

15. I can learn the right foods
    for me.   1 2 3 4 5

16. I can eat ordinary foods.   1 2 3 4 5

17. The foods on my diet are
    good for everyone.   1 2 3 4 5

18. My dietitian and doctor
    really help.   1 2 3 4 5

19. My family and friends will
    help me stick to my diet.   1 2 3 4 5

20. I'll do anything to improve
    my health.   1 2 3 4 5

Appendix VI

Patterns for Exchange Lists
at Three Caloric Levels

I. Pattern for Exchange Lists* 1000 - 1200 kcal

	CHO	PRO	FAT	KCAL
Breakfast				
2 List 1 Starch/Bread	30	6		160
1 List 5 Milk (skim)	12	8	tr	90
Sub Total	42	14	tr	250
Lunch				
2 List 2 Meat (lean)		14	6	110
1 List 1 Starch/Bread	15	3		80
2 List 3 Vegetable	10	4		50
1 Free Vegetable				--
1 List 4 Fruit	15			60
1 List 6 Fat			5	45
Sub Total	40	21	11	345
Dinner				
2 List 2 Meat (medfat)		14	10	150
2 List 1 Starch/Bread	30	6		160
2 List 3 Vegetable	10	4		50
1 Free Vegetable				--
1 List 4 Fruit	15			60
Sub Total	55	24	10	420
H. S.				
1 List 1 Starch/Bread	15	3		80
1 List 5 Milk (Skim)	12	8	tr	90
Sub Total	27	11		170
Grand Total	164	70	21	1185
% kcal	55	24	16	

* Designed for inhospital use. Discharge diets should be individualized for the patient.

II. Pattern for Exchange Lists*   1500 - 1600kcal

	CHO	PRO	FAT	KCAL
Breakfast				
2 List 1 Starch/Bread	30	6		160
1 List 5 Milk (skim)	12	8	tr	90
1 List 6 Fat			5	45
Sub Total	42	14	5	295
Lunch				
3 List 2 Meat (lean)		21	9	165
2 List 1 Starch/Bread	30	6		160
2 List 3 Vegetable	10	4		50
1 List 4 Fruit	15			60
1 List 6 Fat			5	45
Sub Total	55	31	14	480
Dinner				
3 List 2 Meat (medfat)		21	15	225
2 List 1 Starch/Bread	30	6		160
2 List 3 Vegetables	10	4		50
1 List 4 Fruit	15			60
1 List 6 Fat			5	45
1 Free				--
Sub Total	55	31	20	540
H.S.				
1 List 1 Starch/Bread	15	3		80
1 List 5 Milk (skim)	12	8	tr	90
1 List 6 Fat			5	45
Sub Total	27	11	5	215
Grand Total	179	87	44	1530
% kcal	47	23	26	

* Designed for inhospital use. Discharge diets should be individualized for the patient.

III. Pattern for Exchange Lists*   2000 - 2100 kcal

	CHO	PRO	FAT	KCAL
Breakfast				
2 List 1 Starch/Bread	30	6		160
1 List 2 Meat (lean)		7	3	55
1 List 5 Milk (skim)	12	8	tr	90
1 List 6 Fat			5	45
Sub Total	42	21	8	350
A.M.				
1 List 4 Fruit	15			60
1 List 1 Starch/Bread	15	3		80
Sub Total	30	3	0	140
Lunch				
3 List 2 Meat (lean)		21	9	165
2 List 1 Starch/Bread	30	6		160
2 List 3 Vegetable	10	4		50
1 List 4 Fruit	15			60
1 List 6 Fat			5	45
Sub Total	55	31	14	480
P.M.				
1 List 1 Starch/Bread	15	3		80
1 List 5 Milk (skim)	12	8	tr	90
Sub Total	27	11	0	170
Dinner				
3 List 2 Meat (medfat)		21	15	225
2 List 1 Starch/Bread	30	6		160
2 List 3 Vegetable	10	4		50
2 List 4 Fruit	30			120
1 List 6 Fat			5	45
Sub Total	70	31	20	600
H.S.				
2 List 1 Starch/Bread	30	6		160
1 List 5 Milk (skim)	12	8		90
1 List 2 Meat (lean)		7	3	55
1 List 6 Fat			5	45
Sub Total	42	21	8	350
Grand Total	266	118	50	2090
% kcal	51	23	22	

* Designed for inhospital use. Discharge diets should be individualized for the patient.

Appendix VII

Special Menu Plans

Special Menus Plan I
800 kcal - Two Meal Pattern -Three Days

Food	Amount	kcal
Day 1 - Meal 1 (9:30 a.m.)		
Bran Cereal	1/2 cup	76
Blueberries	1/2 cup	40
Milk, skim	1 cup	90
Bagel, dry	1 large	163
Cream Cheese, low calorie	1 Tbsp	30
Strawberry Preserves, low calorie	2 tsp	16
Day 1 - Meal 2 (5:30 p.m.)		
Haddock	3 1/2 oz	141
Potato, baked	1 large	139
Sour Cream, low calorie	1 Tbsp	30
Mixed Vegetables, frozen	1/2 cup	60
Celery Sticks	5	10
Gelatin Dessert w/sweetner	1/2 cup	8
Water/Coffee/Tea/Sweetener		--
Total - Day 1		803

Special Menu Plan I
800 kcal - Two Meal Pattern - Three Days

Food	Amount	kcal
Day 2 - Meal 1		
Grapefruit	1/2 cup	37
Soft Boiled Egg	2	158
Bread, thin sliced	2 slices	98
Margarine, low calorie	2 tsp	35
Grilled Tomatoes	1 medium	20
Milk, skim	1/2 cup	45
Coffee/Tea/Sweetener		--
Day 2 - Meal 2 (5:30 p.m.)		
Chicken without skin	3 1/2 oz	173
Spaghetti (boiled)	1 cup	108
Parmesan Cheese	1 Tbsp	33
Green Beans w/Mushrooms	1/2 cup	29
Shredded Carrots and Cabbage	1/2 cup	25
Mayonnaise, low calorie	1 Tbsp	40
Water/Coffee/Tea/Sweetener		--
Total Day 2		801

Special Menus Plan I
800 kcal - Two Meal Pattern - Three Days

Food	Amount	kcal
Day 3 - Meal 1 (9:30 a.m.)		
Cheese Toast:		
Bread, thin slice	2 slices	98
Cheese, low calorie	2 oz	100
Mustard		--
Yogurt, plain	1/2 cup	75
Sweetener		--
Melon	1/4 cup	25
Strawberries	1/4 cup	15
Milk, skim	6 oz	70
Day 3 - Meal 2 (5:30 p.m.)		
Commercial Low Calorie Entree	1 serving	260
Hearts of Lettuce	1/8 head	15
Low Calorie Dressing	1 Tbsp	30
Ice Cream, low calorie	1/2 cup	100
Water/Tea/Coffee/Sweetener		--
Total - Day 3		788

Meals should be eaten at the hours indicated, nothing but water, tea, coffee or low caloric beverages between meals.

Note: These menus approach nutritional adequacy, additional skim milk would improve the riboflavin and calcium values.

Values from labelled products and Pennington and Church (14th Edition).

Special Menu Plan II
1000-1200 kcal Three Meal Pattern- Three Days
(Home cooked and some convenience foods)

Food	Amount	kcal
Day 1 -Meal 1 (9:30 a.m.)		
Bran Cereal	1/3 cup	71
Blueberries	1/2 cup	41
Egg, fried	1 medium	83
Whole Wheat Toast	2 slices	120
Margarine	1 tsp	35
Milk, skim	1 cup	90
Coffee/Tea/Sweetener	--	-
Day 1 - Meal 2		
Chicken Salad	1/2 cup	150
Whole Wheat Roll	1	160
Banana Pudding Pop	1	94
Water/Coffee/Tea/Sweetener	--	-
Day 1 - Meal 3		
Lima Bean and Ham Casserole	1/2 cup	220
Corn	1 ear	114
Sliced Tomato Salad	1/2 cup	20
Watermelon	1 cup	52
Water/Tea/Coffee/Sweetener	--	-
Total for Day 1		1250

Special Menu Plan II
1000-1200 kcal Three Meal Pattern- Three Days
(Home cooked and some convenience foods)

Food	Amount	kcal
Day 2 -Meal 1		
Banana	1 small	105
Bran/raisin flakes	1/2 cup	87
Biscuits	2 small	130
Margarine	1 tsp	35
Low Calorie Jelly	2 tsps	16
Milk, skim	1 cup	90
Coffee/Tea/Sweetener	--	-
Day 2 - Meal 2		
Chef's Salad made with		
Hard Boiled Egg	1/2	40
Turkey, white meat	2 oz	120
Raw Vegetables		--
Low Calorie Dressing	1 Tbsp	30
Rye Crisp Crackers	2	60
Apple with skin	1 medium	81
Water/Coffee/Tea/Sweetener	--	-
Day 2 - Meal 3		
Low Calorie Entree, frozen	1 as packed	300
Broccoli	1/2 cup	20
Green Salad	1/2 cup	25
Grapes, seedless	1/2 cup	48
Water/Coffee/Tea/Sweetener	--	-
Total for Day 2		1187

Special Menu Plan II
1000-1200 kcal Three Meal Pattern - Three Days
(Home cooked and some commercial foods)

Food	Amount	kcal
Day 3 -Meal 1		
Prunes, canned in heavy syrup	5	90
Puffed Wheat	1 cup	50
Bran Muffin	1	112
Margarine, low calorie	1 tsp	15
Milk, Skim	1 cup	90
Coffee/Tea/Sweetener	-	-
Day 3 - Meal 2		
Tuna Noodle Casserole, frozen	1 cup	200
Tomato Salad	1/2 cup	25
Raw Pineapple	1 cup	77
Water/Coffee/Tea/Sweetener	-	-
Day 3 - Meal 3		
Chili Con Carne with Beans	3 1/2 oz	133
Fresh Carrots (steamed)	5	25
Whole Wheat Roll	1/2 small	90
Tossed Salad	1/2 cup	13
Low Calorie Dressing	1 Tbsp	30
Low Calorie Vanilla Pudding Pop	1 serving	67
Water/Coffee/Tea/Sweetener	--	-
Total Day 3		1017

Special Menu Plan III
1200-1400 kcal - Three Meal Pattern - Three Days
(Restaurant and Fast Food Based)[1,2]

Food	Amount	kcal
Day I - Meal 1		
Egg McMuffin	1	327
Coffee/Tea/Sweetener	-	-
Day I - Meal 2		
Cheese Pizza (10 inch)	1/2	359
Green Salad	1/2 cup	25
Dressing	2 tsp	50
Low Calorie Beverage	8 oz	--
Day I - Meal 3		
Baked Chicken, no skin	1/4 chicken	205
Potato Steak Fries	3/4 cup	121
Peas, Green	2/3 cup	71
Green Salad	1/2 cup	25
Dressing	2 tsp	50
Water/Coffee/Tea/Sweetener	--	-
Total Day I		1233

Special Menu Plan III
1200-1400 kcal - Three Meal Pattern - Three Days

Food	Amount	kcal
Day 2 - Meal 1		
Grapefruit, Fresh	1/2	37
Egg, Fried	1 medium	83
Toast, Dry	1 slice	64
Margarine	1 tsp	35
Coffee/Tea/Sweetener	--	-
Day 2 - Meal 2		
Soup, Vegetable	1 cup	75
Fruit Salad Plate:		
Assorted Fresh Fruit	1 cup	180
Cottage Cheese	1/2 cup	117
Crackers	2	60
Coffee/Tea/Sweetener	--	-
Day 2 - Meal 3		
Steak, Broiled	3 oz	235
Potato, Baked	1 medium	95
Sour Cream	1 tsp	50
Green Beans	1/2 cup	35
Tomato Salad, no dressing	1/2 cup	30
Milk, Whole	1 cup	150
Total Day 2		1190

Special Menu Plan III
1200-1400 kcal - Three Meal Pattern - Three Days
(Restaurant and Fast Food Based) [1,2]

	Amount	kcal
Day 3 - Meal 1		
Corn Flakes	1 cup	105
Banana, Fresh	1 medium	120
Doughnut, Raised Yeast	1 piece	124
Milk, Whole	1 cup	150
Coffee/Iced Tea/Sweetener	--	-
Day 3 - Meal 2		
Hamburger, Fast Food	1	290
Soft Ice Cream	1 small	170
Coffee/iced Tea/Sweetener	--	-
Day 3 - Meal 3		
Liver, Fried	3 1/2 oz	229
Mashed Potato	1/2 cup	94
Fried Onions	1/3 cup	80
Cole Slaw	1 cup	82
Sliced Peaches, Canned (1/2 peach with juice)	1/2 peach	66
Water/Coffee/Tea/Sweetener	--	-
Total Day 3		1510

[1] Many of these values are taken from restaurant chain publications.
[2] These menus are high in sodium, saturated fat and cholesterol.

Appendix VIII

Sample Menus
with Various Energy Levels

For 1000-1400 kcal Menus,
see Special Menus II, Days 1, 2, 3
and
Special Menus III, Days 1, 2, 3

Sample Menu - 2400 kcal

Food	Amount
Breakfast	
Canadian bacon	1 oz
Pancakes, small	3
Syrup, low calorie	2 Tbsp
Milk, 2%	1 cup
Lunch	
Pizza with cheese	1 piece
Tossed salad	1 cup
Dressing (Italian)	1 Tbsp
Apple, medium	1
Milk, 2%	1 cup
Snack	
Yogurt, low fat, plain	1 cup
Banana, medium	1
Dinner	
Chicken, baked	3 oz
Potato, boiled, small	2
Margarine	2 tsp
Cole slaw (mayonnaise)	1/2 cup
Peach (fresh), medium	1
Milk, 2%	1 cup
Snack	
Peanut butter	2 Tbsp
Crackers (medium)	6
Milk, 2%	1 cup

Total kilocalories - 2347

	Grams	% kcal
Carbohydrate	290	48
Protein	123	21
Fat	84	31
Fiber	32	

Sample Menu - 2600 kcal

Food	Amount
Breakfast	
Bran flakes	1 cup
Whole wheat toast, slices	2
Margarine	2 tsp
Milk, 2%	1 cup
Lunch	
Tossed salad	1 cup
French dressing	1 Tbsp
Orange, medium	1
Oatmeal cookies	2
Milk, 2%	1 cup
Snack	
Yogurt, non-fat	8 oz
Banana, medium	1
Dinner	
Roast beef	3 oz
Baked potato, small	1
Sour cream	2 Tbsp
Tossed salad	1 cup
Italian dressing	1 Tbsp
Broccoli, fresh, cooked	1 cup
Fresh pineapple cubes	1/2 cup
Milk, 2%	1 cup
Snack	
Crackers, medium	6
Milk, 2%	1 cup

Total kilocalories - 2652

	Grams	% kcal
Carbohydrate	338	49
Protein	139	20
Fat	93	30
Fiber	46	

Appendix IX

Sample Menu for Teenage Female
Sample Menus for Pregnancy
and Lactation

Sample Menu - 2200 kcal Teenage Female

Food	Amount
Breakfast	
Whole wheat cereal	3/4 cup
Whole wheat toast, sliced	2
Margarine	1 tsp
Milk, skim	1 cup
Lunch	
Turkey, white meat	3 oz
Multi grain bread, sliced	2
Fresh fruit	1 piece
Milk, skim	1 cup
Diet Mayonnaise	2 tsp
Snack	
Non fat yogurt, plain	1 cup
Dinner	
Baked or broiled fish	3 oz
Rice	3/4 cup
Cooked vegetable	1/2 cup
Tossed salad	1 cup
Salad dressing	1 Tbsp
Whole wheat roll	1
Margarine	2 tsp
Fresh fruit	1 piece
Milk, skim	1 cup
Snack	
Low fat cheese	1 oz
Whole wheat crackers	6
Milk, skim	1 cup

Total kilocalories -- 2140

	Grams	% kcal
Carbohydrate	288	54
Protein	141	26
Fat	49	20
Fiber	28	

Sample Menu for Pregnancy and Lactation 2300 kcal

Food	Amount
Breakfast	
Shredded wheat biscuit	1
Scrambled eggs	2 eggs
Margarine	2 tsp
Milk, 2%	1 cup
Lunch	
Hamburger, meat	3 oz
Bun, small	1
Tossed Salad	1 cup
Dressing, low calorie	1 Tbsp
Strawberries	1/2 cup
Milk, 2%	1 cup
Dinner	
Chicken, baked, small	1/4
Rice, boiled	3/4 cup
Roll, small	1
Margarine	1 tsp
Broccoli	1/2 cup
Pear, fresh	1
Pound cake, small piece	1
Milk, 2%	1 cup
H.S. Snack	
Peanut butter	1 Tbsp
Saltines	4
Milk, 2%	1 cup

Total kilocalories - 2267

	Grams	% kcal
Carbohydrate	230	40
Protein	123	21
Fat	97	38
Fiber	21	

Sample Menu for Pregnancy and Lactation 2500 kcal

Food	Amount
Breakfast	
Special K	1 cup
Pancakes, medium	2
Margarine	2 tsp
Imitation syrup	1 oz
Milk, 2%	1 cup
Snack	
Non-fat yogurt	3/4 cup
Apple, medium	1
Lunch	
Tuna Sandwich	
Tuna	3 oz
Whole wheat bread, sliced	2
Carrot/celery sticks	4 each
Orange, small	1
Potato chips	10
Milk, 2%	1 cup
Dinner	
Baked fish	4 oz
Tartar sauce	1 Tbsp
French fries	10
Green beans	1 cup
Roll, small	1
Margarine	1 tsp
Milk, 2%	1 cup
H.S. Snack	
Graham crackers	2
Apple, small	1
Milk, 2%	1 cup
Additional Snack	
Bread, sliced	1
Cheese	1 oz
Milk, 2%	1 cup

Total kilocalories - 2484

	Grams	% kcal
Carbohydrate	289	46
Protein	144	23
Fat	88	21
Fiber	27	

```
        Sample Menu for Pregnancy and Lactation
                       2800 kcal
```

Food	Amount
Breakfast	
Bran flakes, 40%	3/4 cup
Egg, poached	1
Whole wheat bread, sliced	2
Margarine	2 tsp
Milk, 2%	1 cup
Lunch	
Turkey sandwich	
turkey	3 oz
whole wheat bread, sliced	2
mayonnaise	2 tsp
lettuce/tomato (leaf/slice)	1
Apple, medium	1
Milk, 2%	1 cup
Dinner	
Roast Beef	3 oz
Potato, baked, medium	1
Margarine	2 tsp
Carrots, cooked	2/3 cup
Roll	1
Margarine	1 tsp
Cantaloupe, medium	1/4
Milk, 2%	1 cup
H.S. Snack	
Milk, 2%	1 cup
Cheese	1 oz
Saltines	6
Additional Snack	
Peanut butter	1 Tbsp
Saltines	6
Milk, 2%	1 cup

Total kilocalories - 2741

	Grams	% kcal
Carbohydrate	262	38
Protein	145	21
Fat	127	41

Appendix X

Sample Menus for High Fiber, High Carbohydrate

Sample Menu for High Fiber, High Carbohydrate
1100 kilocalories.

Food	Amount
Breakfast	
Oat bran flakes	3/4 cup
Whole wheat toast	1 slice
Margarine, diet	1 tsp
Milk, skim	1/2 cup
Lunch	
Bean soup	1 cup
Rye crisp	4
Salad green	1 cup
Carrots, raw	1/4 cup
Zucchini, raw	1/4 cup
Bean sprouts	1/4 cup
Cabbage, raw	1/4 cup
Italian dressing, diet	1 Tbsp
Cottage cheese, low fat	1/4 cup
Apple, small	1
Dinner	
Flounder, baked	4 oz
Pasta, cooked	1 cup
Pasta sauce	1/2 cup
Brussel sprouts	1/2 cup
Cantaloupe, small	1/4
Milk, skim	1 cup

Total kilocalories - 1111

	Grams	% kcal
Carbohydrate	164	57
Protein	86	30
Fat	16	13
Fiber	19	

t et al.* 209*

Sample Menu for High Fiber, High Carbohydrate
1500 kilocalories

Food	Amount
Breakfast	
Shredded wheat	1 cup
Whole wheat toast, sliced	2
Margarine	2 tsp
Milk, skim	1/2 cup
Lunch	
Turkey	2 oz
Whole wheat bread,	2 slices
Mayonnaise	1 tsp
Lettuce	1 cup
Tomato, small	1
French dressing, diet	1 Tbsp
Broccoli	1 cup
Garbanzo beans	1/2 cup
Grapes	12
Dinner	
Fish, baked	3 oz
Brown rice	3/4 cup
Green beans	1 cup
Margarine	2 tsp
Pickled beet salad	1/2 cup
Orange/grapefruit sections	1 1/2 cups

Total kilocalories - 1488

	Grams	% kcal
Carbohydrate	217	56
Protein	91	24
Fat	35	20
Fiber	45	

Sample Menu High Fiber, High Carbohydrate
1600 kilocalories

Food	Amount
Breakfast	
Oatmeal	1 1/2 cups
Whole wheat toast	2 slices
Margarine	1 tsp
Milk, skim	1 cup
Lunch	
Salad	
Mixed greens	1/2 cup
Cauliflower, raw	1/2 cup
Zucchini, raw	1/2 cup
Broccoli, raw	1/2 cup
Carrots, raw	1/2 cup
Garbanzo beans	1/2 cup
Cheese, low fat	1 oz
Tomato, sliced, medium	1
Italian dressing	2 Tbsp
Apple, small with skin	1
Bran muffin	1
Dinner	
Chicken, baked	3 oz
Sweet potato, baked (small)	1
Corn	1/2 cup
Green beans	1/2 cup
Broccoli spears	4
Rye bread	1 slice
Margarine	1 Tbsp
Graham crackers	2
Snack	
Yogurt, low-fat, plain	1 cup
Strawberries	3/4 cup
Sweetner	1 packet

Total kilocalories - 1597

	Grams	% kcal
Carbohydrate	218	52
Protein	91	22
Fat	47	26
Fiber	46	

Sample Menu High Fiber, High Carbohydrate
1800 kilocalories

Food	Amount
Breakfast	
Bran muffin	1
Breakfast yogurt	
Yogurt, plain	1 cup
Pineapple, crushed, unsweetened	1/2 cup
Sugar substitute	1 packet
Grape nuts cereal	1/4 cup
Lunch	
Turkey, sliced	1 oz
Whole wheat bread	2 slices
Tomato	2 slices
Navy bean soup	1 cup
Whole wheat crackers	4
Asparagus salad	4 spears
Dinner	
Spaghetti, whole wheat	1 cup
Tomato sauce	1/2 cup
Ground beef, lean	2 oz
Summer squash, steamed	1 cup
Tossed salad with lettuce, cucumber, celery, green pepper, cauliflower, carrots	1 1/2 cup
French dressing	1 Tbsp
Banana, small	1
Snack	
"Alba 77" milkshake	1
Bran muffin	1

Total kilocalories - 1769

Carbohydrate	250	54
Protein	88	19
Fat	55	27
Fiber	30	

Appendix XI

Caloric Values of Selected Foods

Caloric Value of Selected Foods from:

Ref: Calories and Weight, The USDA Pocket Guide Home
and Garden Bulletin 153. U.S. Dept. of Agriculture,
Washington, D.C., 1972.

BEVERAGES   Calories
(Calories from these foods are from table
sugar) (Not including milk and fruit juice)

Fruit Drinks:
Cranberry juice cocktail, 1/2 cup   80
Grape drink, 1/2 cup   70
Lemonade, frozen concentrate, sweetened, ready-
  to-serve, 1/2 cup (regular)   55
Orange juice-apricot juice drink, 1/2 cup   60

Carbonated Beverages:
Cola-type, 12 oz can   145
Fruit flavors, 10-13% sugar, 12 oz can   170
Gingerale, 12 oz can   115
Root beer, 12 oz can   150
(Check the label of "diet" drinks for the number
  of calories provided)

Alcoholic Beverages:
Beer, 3.6% alcohol, 8 oz glass   100
                  12 oz can or bottle   150
Whiskey, gin, rum, vodka
  80-proof, 1 1/2 oz   95
  86-proof, 1 1/2 oz   105
  90-proof, 1 1/2 oz   110
  100-proof, 1 1/2 oz   125
Wines, table (Chablis, claret, Rhine,
  burgundy, etc.), 3 1/2 oz   85
  (kcal will be from sugars)
Wines, dessert (muscatel, port, sherry,
  Tokay, etc.), 3 1/2 oz   140
  (kcal will be from sugars)

BREAD AND CEREALS
Cracked Wheat, 18 slices per pound loaf, 1 slice   65
Raisin, 18 slices per pound loaf, 1 slice   65
White, regular slice, 18 per pound, 1 slice   70
       thin slice, 22 per pound, 1 slice   55
Whole Wheat, 16 slices per pound loaf, 1 slice   65

	Calories
Rice, puffed, 1 oz (about 2 cups)	115
Wheat, puffed, 1 oz (about 1 7/8 cups)	105
shredded, plain, 1 oz (1 large biscuit or 1/2 cup bite-size)	100
flakes, 1 oz (about 1 cup)	100

Biscuits, Muffins, Rolls:
Baking powder biscuit

home recipe, 2 inch diameter, one	105
mix, 2 inch diameter, one	100
Muffin plain, 3 inch diameter, one	120
blueberry, 2 3/8 inch diameter, one	110
bran, 2 5/8 inch diameter, one	105

Roll

hamburger or frankfurter, (10 per pound), one	120
hard, round, or rectangular, (9 per pound), one	155
sweet, pan, (11 per pound), one	135

Cracker

butter, about 2 inch diameter, one	15
graham, 2 1/2 inch square, two	55
matzo, 6 inch diameter piece, one	80
oyster, ten	35
saltines, 1 7/8 inch square, four	50

Doughnut

Cake-type, plain, 3 1/4 inch diameter (1 1/2 oz), one	165
Yeast-leavened, raised, 3 3/4 inch diameter, (1 1/2 oz), one	175
Danish pastry, plain, 4 1/2 inch diameter, one	275

Cakes

Angelcake, 2 1/2 inch sector of 9 3/4 inch round cake	135
Chocolate cake, with chocolate icing, 1 3/4 inch sector of 9 inch round layer cake	235
Plain cake, with chocolate icing, 1 3/4 inch sector of 9 inch round layer cake	240
Pound cake, old fashion, 3 1/2 inch square	140

Other Grain Products:

Corn grits, degermed, cooked, 3/4 cup	95
Macaroni, cooked with cheese, home recipe, 1/2 cup	215
Noodles, cooked, 3/4 cup	150

Rice, cooked, instant, 3/4 cup 135
Spaghetti, cooked in tomato sauce,
    with cheese, 3/4 cup 195

CANDIES
Chocolate, milk, sweetened, with almonds,
    1 oz bar 150
Fudge, vanilla or chocolate, plain, 1 oz 115
Hard Candy, three or four 3/4 inch diameter
    candy balls (1 ounce) 110

OTHER SWEETS
Honey, 1 tablespoon 65
Jam, preserves, 1 tablespoon 55
Jelly, marmalade, 1 tablespoon 50
Molasses, 1 tablespoon 50
Syrup, table blends, 1 tablespoon 55
Sugar, white, granulated or brown (packed),
    1 teaspoon 15

COOKIES
Chocolate chip, 2 1/3 inch cookie, 1/2 inch
    thick, one 50
Vanilla wafer, 1 3/4 inch cookie 20

PIES:
Apple, 1/8 of 9 inch pie 300
Lemon meringue, 1/8 of 9 inch pie 270
Pumpkin, 1/8 of 9 inch pie 240

OTHER DESSERTS
Brownie, with nuts, 1 3/4 inch square, 7/8 inch
    thick 90
Gelatin
    plain, 1/2 cup 70
    with fruit, 1/2 cup 80
Ice cream, plain, regular (about 10% fat),
    1/2 cup 130
Ice milk, soft serve, 1/2 cup 135
Pudding, chocolate, from a mix, 1/2 cup 160
Sherbet, 1/2 cup 130

FATS, OILS, CREAMS AND RELATED PRODUCTS

Fats and Oils:
Butter or margarine, 1 tablespoon 100
Margarine, whipped, soft, tub, 1 tablespoon 100

Salad oil, 1 tablespoon	120
Salad dressings, regular	
blue cheese, 1 tablespoon	75
Italian, 1 tablespoon	70
mayonnaise, 1 tablespoon	100
salad dressing, commercial	
plain (mayonnaise-type), 1 tablespoon	55
Salad dressings, low calorie	
French, 1 tablespoon	20
Cream, half-and-half (milk and cream),	
1 tablespoon	20
Whipped topping, pressurized, 1 tablespoon	10
Creamers, powdered, 1 teaspoon	10

MEAT, POULTRY, FISH, EGGS, DRIED BEANS
AND PEAS, NUTS

Beef:	
Chili con carne, canned	
with beans, 1/2 cup	170
without beans, 1/2 cup	240
Hamburger, broiled, panbroiled, or sauteed	
regular, 3 oz	245
lean, 3 oz	185
Oven roast, cooked, without bone, cuts relatively	
fat such as rib	
lean and fat, 3 oz	375
lean only, 3 oz	205
Steak, broiled, without bone	
such as sirloin	
lean and fat, 3 oz	330
lean only, 3 oz	175
such as round	
lean and fat, 3 oz	220
Pork:	
Bacon, broiled or fried, crisp, 2 medium slices	85
Chop, broiled without bone, lean and fat, 3 oz	335
Ham, cured, cooked, without bone, lean	
only, 3 oz	160
Sausage:	
Bologna, 2 ounces, (2 very thin slices, 4 1/2	
inch diameter)	170
Pork, link, cooked, four, 4 inch links (4 oz	
uncooked)	250
Salami, 2 oz (two 4 1/2 inch diameter slices)	175
Frankfurter, cooked, (8 per pound), one	170
Boiled ham, 2 ounces, (2 very thin 6 1/4 x 4	
inch slices)	135

Poultry:
```
Chicken, roasted (no skin), breast, one half        140
Turkey, roasted (no skin)
  light meat, 3 oz                                  135
  dark meat, 3 oz                                   160
```
Fish and Shellfish":
```
Haddock, breaded, fried, 3 oz (4 x 2 1/2 x
  1/2 inch)                                         140
Salmon, broiled or baked, 3 oz                      155
Shrimp, canned, 27 medium (3 oz)                    100
Tunafish, canned in oil, drained, 1/2 cup, 3 oz     170
```
Eggs:
```
Hard or soft cooked, large, one                      80
```
Nuts:
```
Peanuts, 2 tablespoons                              105
Peanut Butter, 1 tablespoon                          95
Walnuts, chopped, 2 tablespoons                     105
```

MILK AND CHEESE

Milk:
```
Buttermilk, 1 cup                                   100
Condensed, sweetened, undiluted, 1/2 cup            490
Evaporated, whole, undiluted, 1/2 cup               170
Lowfat, 2% fat, nonfat milk solids added, 1 cup     125
Skim, 1 cup                                          85
Whole, 1 cup                                        150
Yogurt, made from skim milk, 1 cup                  125
```
Cheese:
```
American, process, 1 oz                             105
Cheddar, natural, 1 oz                              115
Cottage, creamed, 1 cup                             250
```

SNACKS AND OTHER "EXTRAS"

```
French fries, fresh, ten 3 1/2 x 1/4 inch pieces    215
Pizza, plain cheese, 5 1/3 inch sector of 13 3/4
  inch pie                                          155
Popcorn, large-kernel, popped with oil and salt,
  1 cup                                              40
Potato chips, ten 1 3/4 x 2 1/2 inch chips          115
Pretzel sticks, five 3 1/8 inches long               60
Tomato catsup or chili sauce, 1 tablespoon           15
```

VEGETABLES (RAW)
```
Cabbage, coleslaw with mayonnaise, 1/2 cup           85
```

Lettuce
  leaves, large, two   5
  shredded or chopped, 1/2 cup   5

VEGETABLES (COOKED, CANNED, FROZEN)
Beans
  green lima, 1/2 cup   90
  snap, green, wax, or yellow, 1/2 cup   15
Beets, diced, sliced, or small whole, 1/2 cup   30
Broccoli, stalks, three 4 1/2 to 5 inch   25
Corn
  on cob, one 5 inch ear   70
  cream-style, 1/2 cup   105
Peas, green, 1/2 cup   65
Potatoes
  baked, 2 1/3 inch diameter, 4 3/4 inch long   145
  hash-browned, 1/2 cup   175
  mashed, milk and fat added, 1/2 cup   100
  salad, made with mayonnaise or French dressing
    and eggs, 1/2 cup   180
Sweetpotatoes
  baked in skin, 2 inch diameter, 5 inches long   160

FRUITS (RAW)
Apples, 2 3/4 inch diameter, one   80
Avocado, Florida varieties, 16 ounce, 1/2   205
Bananas, 6 to 7 inch (about 1/3 pound)   85
Cantaloupe, 5 inch, 1/2   80
Dates, "fresh" and dried, pitted, cut, 1/2 cup   245
Grapefruit, 3 3/4 inch fruit, 1/2   50
Grapes, seedless, (Flame, Tokay, etc.), 1/2 cup   55
Oranges, 2 5/8 inch diameter   65
Pineapple, diced, 1/2 cup   40
Raisins, packed, 1/2 cup   240
Strawberries, 1/2 cup   30
Watermelon, 2 pound wedge   110

FRUITS (COOKED, CANNED, OR FROZEN)
Applesauce, sweetened, 1/2 cup   115
Apricots, dried, cooked, unsweetened, fruit and
  juice, 1/2 cup   105
Fruit cocktail, canned in heavy syrup, 1/2 cup   95
Peaches
  canned in water, 1/2 cup   40
  canned in heavy syrup, 1/2 cup   100
Pineapple, canned, crushed, tidbits or chunks
  in heavy syrup, 1/2 cup   95

Prunes, dried, cooked
   unsweetened, fruit and liquid, 1/2 cup   125
    sweetened, fruit and liquid, 1/2 cup   205
Strawberries, frozen, sweetened, sliced, 1/2 cup 105

FRUIT JUICES
Apple, canned, 1/2 cup   60
Orange
   fresh, 1/2 cup   55
   canned, unsweetened, 1/2 cup   60
   frozen concentrate, ready-to-serve, 1/2 cup 55
Prune, canned, 1/2 cup   100

Appendix XII

Resource Information

Resource Information

Professional organizations provide information for their members and the public. For example:

American Association of Diabetes Educators
500 N. Michigan Avenue
Chicago, IL 60611, (312) 661-1700

The American Dietetic Association
216 W. Jackson Blvd., Suite 800
Chicago, IL 60606, (312) 899-0040
    Members only (800) 877-1600

Government Agencies can offer materials, services and referrals. For Example:

State Health Departments

National Diabetes Information Clearinghouse
Box NDIC
Bethesda, MD 20205 , (202) 842-7630

Voluntary Health Associations, local, state and national can provide information and services. Many state organizations have toll-free numbers. For example:

American Diabetes Association
American Cancer Association
American Heart Association.

Glossary

Additives — see food terms

Adipose — see body weight terms

Adiposity — see body weight terms

Algae — see carbohydrates, fiber

Alternate Eating Patterns

Vegetarian: Pattern that relies primarily on plant foods.

Lacto-Ovo-Vegetarian: Uses eggs and milk but excludes animal and marine flesh from the diet.

Vegan: Pure vegetarian, uses only plant foods.

Amino acids — see proteins

Anabolism — see energy

Anorexia nervosa — see eating disorders

Arachdonic acid — see lipids

Aspartame — see nutritive sweeteners

Autointoxication — see questionable nutrition practices and approaches

Average weight — see body weight and wt/ht tables

Basal metabolism — see energy

Basic Four Food Group Guide — see nutritional needs and food intake

Basic Seven Food Group Guide — see nutritional needs and food intake

Biological value — see protein

Blood glucose, self-monitoring — see diabetes terms

Blood lipids — see lipids

Blood sugar — see diabetes terms

Body Weight and Weight/Height Tables

Average Weight: Weight per height tables before 1942 were "average" weights per height. Data for the tables were compiled from life insurance companies' information on applicants for life insurance policies. Average data and the tables reflected an increase in weight per height with age.

Ideal Body Weight: This term was used by The Metropolitan Life Insurance Company in 1942-43 in describing weights of men and women per heights. The table published was based on the premise that "ideal body weight" is below the average for the insured population that was examined. The tables were based on 1913 and 1932 mortality studies done by the Society of Actuaries and the Association of Life Insurance Medical Directors and on studies published by The Metropolitan Life Insurance Company in 1937 and 1939.

Desirable Weight: In 1959 Metropolitan presented revised tables called "Desirable Weight Tables." The figures were based on data from the 1959 Build and Blood Pressure Study of the Society of Actuaries and the Medical Directors. The "desirable" weights in the tables indicated the weight associated with the lowest mortality of insured people. Weights below the average were again considered most "desirable" for long life. Both the 1942-43 and the 1959 Metropolitan tables were divided into three body frame units, small, medium and large, but no directions were given for determining frame size. No weight change after age 25 was considered "ideal" or "desirable." Weights were given as "ordinarily dressed" in the 1942-43 tables, and with "indoor clothing" in 1959. Heights in both tables were given with shoes. A Suggested Weight for Height table was published in the sixties by Hathaway and Foard from a USDA study of previous published data.

Recommended Weights in Relation to Height: Table was published in 1973 by the Fogarty International Center Conference on Obesity. It was an adaptation of the Metropolitan Tables of heights without shoes and weights without clothing. Weights per height were given both as average and as a range. The mean weights of these tables were used in the 1980 RDAs.

Desirable Weights: Hanes data of 1971-1974 were used as the basis for tables of "desirable weights." Desirable weights were defined as mean weights between ages 20-29.

Latest Height/Weight Tables: Are from Metropolitan Life Insurance Co. (1983) based on a Build Study of 1979 (Society of Actuaries and Association of Life Insurance Medical Directors). Figures for weight are those associated with lowest mortality. People with serious illnesses were excluded. Methods to measure body frame size were included. Weights per height are somewhat larger than in the 1959 charts. No descriptive terms, e.g., "ideal" or "desirable" are given on the tables.

Body Weight Terms:

Adipose Tissue: Connective tissue or spaces within tissues containing masses of fat cells.

Adiposity: Excessive accumulation of fat in the body.

Obesity: Excessive fat accumulation in the body. An abnormal amount of fat. Term frequently employed with a body weight of 20-30% over average weight per height (20% for men, 28-30% for women) or when 20 to 30% of the body weight is fat.

Overweight: An ill-defined category of body weight. It represents a continuum of weight per height above average and below obese.

Underweight: Usually described as 15% below desirable weight. It actually is the absence of necessary body fat.

Bulimia — see eating disorders
Bulimia, diabetic — see eating disorders

calorie-see energy
Calorie-see energy
Carbohydrates: One of the three main classes of energy nutrients. They are chemical compounds found in plant and animal tissues. Plants produce carbohydrates through the process of photosynthesis, animals form them during metabolism. Carbohydrates are generally classed as yielding 4 kcal/gm, although there is a variation in the caloric value of individual carbohydrates.

Carbohydrate Classification:

1. *Monosaccharides*: also called "simple sugars" because they contain one sugar (saccharide) unit. *Glucose* (also

know as *dextrose*), *fructose* and *galactose* are the best known sugars in this class. They are hexoses because they contain 6 carbon atoms.

2. *Disaccharides*: also called "double sugars" because they contain two saccharide units. The two monosaccharide units in a disaccharide may be the same or different. The most common sugars in this class are *sucrose, maltose* and *lactose*.

3. *Polysaccharides*: are large compounds containing many saccharide units. Although they contain monosaccharide units, they are not sweet, so they are usually referred to as complex carbohydrates or starches rather than sugars. Functionally, polysaccharides are classed as structural or non-structural. The *structural* group includes *cellulose, hemicellulose*, and *some pectins*. The *non-structural polysaccharides* are *starch* (in plants), *glycogen* (starch in animals), as well as *gums, mucilages*, and *algae*.

4. *Oligosaccharides*: a class of carbohydrates frequently used to designate those carbohydrates with *few saccharide units*. There does not seem to be a universal demarcation concerning the number of sugar units present for a carbohydrate to be included in this class. Therefore, the classifications vary as follows:

System 1

Class	Saccharide Units
Monosaccharides	1
Disaccharides	2
Oligosaccharides	3-6
Polysaccharides	more than 6

System 2

Monosaccharides	1
Oligosaccharides	2-10
Polysaccharides	more than 10

Sugar Alcohols: *Sorbitol, mannitol* and *xylitol* are three of the most common naturally occurring sugar alcohols. Sorbitol and mannitol are related to the hexoses (6 carbon sugars) and xylitol is related to the pentoses (5 carbon sugars). Sugar alcohols are not metabolized like sugar in the body, but they contribute essentially the same amount of energy, 4 kcal per gram. They have a sweet taste and are used as substitute sweeteners in food products. The following chart illustrates the most common dietary sources of sugar alcohols:

Polysaccharides	Disaccharides	Monosaccharides	Sugar Alcohols
starch (plants)-------maltose---------glucose------------sorbitol
glycogen-------------maltose---------glucose------------sorbitol
(animal starch)

	lactose-----------glucose------------sorbitol
	(only from
	milk) and
	galactose
	sucrose---------glucose------------sorbitol
	(cane and
	beet sugar, and
	fruits and
	vegetables) fructose-----------mannitol

Carbohydrates, classification — see carbohydrates
Catabolism — see energy
Cellulose — see carbohydrates, fiber
Cellulosic — see fiber
Chelation therapy — see questionable nutrition practices and approaches
Cholesterol — see lipids
Cholesterol altered food — see food terms
Cholesterol esters — see lipids, blood lipids
Chylomicrons — see lipids, blood lipids
Colonic irrigation — see questionable nutrition practices and approaches
Complex carbohydrates — see carbohydrates
Complex proteins — see proteins
Complimentary proteins — see proteins
Condensed milk, sweetened — see food terms

Corn syrup — see nutritive sweeteners
Crude fiber — see fiber
Cytoxic testing — see questionable nutrition practices and approaches

Dawn phenomenon — see diabetes terms
Desirable Weight — see body weight and wt/ht tables
Dextrose — see carbohydrate, nutritive sweeteners
DHA, docosahexanenoic acid — see lipids
Diabetes Terms:

> *Glycosylated Hemoglobin*: When hyperglycemia is sustained for a period of time, the sugar content of hemoglobin (HbA_{1c}, glycosylated Hbg) increases. The attachment of glucose to hemoglobin remains until the red blood cell is degraded. Measurement of glycosylated hemoglobin therefore reflects glycemic control over the previous six to eight weeks.

> *Blood Glucose Self-Monitoring*: *HBGM* — home blood glucose monitoring. Two techniques can be used: (1) a drop of capillary blood (from finger) is placed on a reagent pad at the end of a strip and the resulting color visually matched to a color chart or (2) the color is read by a reflectance meter that provides a read-out from the reagent strip.

> *Hyperglycemia*: Abnormal high levels of glucose in blood.

> *Hypoglycemia*: Abnormal diminished levels of glucose in blood.

> *Euglycemia or Normoglycemia*: a good or normal level of glucose in the blood.

> *Preprandial Blood Sugar*: measurement of blood glucose taken before a meal.

> *Postprandial Blood Sugar*: measurement of blood glucose taken after a meal.

> *Ketosis — Ketoacidosis*: With an insufficiency of insulin there is increased mobilization and break down of fatty acids from the tissues which results in the production of ketone bodies. Lack of insulin also halts the utilization of ketones by the tissues. Both of these events result in the accumula-

tion in the blood of ketones. The ketones increase the acid load of the body causing metabolic acidosis and a life threatening fall in body pH unless insulin is provided. Higher than normal levels of ketones in the blood and urine are known as ketonemia and ketonuria. Three substances are collectively termed *ketone bodies*. They are *acetoacetic acid*, *beta-hydroxy butyric acid* and *acetone*.

Insulin: is a polypeptide consisting of two chains of amino acids which are linked together. It is produced by the beta cells in the Islets of Langerhans of the pancreas, and its secretion is stimulated by high blood glucose. It serves an important role not only in carbohydrate metabolism but is also necessary for glycogen storage, fatty acid synthesis, amino acid uptake and protein synthesis. This anabolic hormone activity is evident in liver, fat, muscle and other tissues.

Glucagon: is a polypeptide consisting of a single chain of amino acids. It is produced by the alpha cells of the Islets of Langerhans of the pancreas. Its secretion is stimulated by low blood sugar. In the tissues affected by insulin and glucagon the two hormones have an antagonistic effect. Whereas insulin is necessary for carbohydrate uptake and protein and fat synthesis, glucagon increases glycogen breakdown and inhibits its synthesis. It also increases the degradation of lipids to fatty acids and glycerol.

Blood Sugar: is glucose, a simple sugar resulting from ingestion of foods, the breakdown of body glycogen or synthesis from non-carbohydrate sources — amino acids and glycerol.

Glycemic Index: A rating system for foods based on their effect on blood glucose in comparison to the blood glucose response to a measured amount of glucose.

Dawn Phenomenon: A term used to describe a rise in blood glucose levels in the early morning hours (dawn) which is not preceded by hypoglycemia or by decreasing insulin levels. The reason for this early morning hyperglycemia is unknown. It has been reported to occur in both NIDDM and IDDM subjects as well as in normal subjects.

Somogyi Effect: Rebound hyperglycemia. Periods of hypoglycemia during the night which may be insulin-induced bring about a hormonal response which can be an over-response or "rebound" effect to the body's need for glucose. The result is morning hyperglycemia with accompanying glycosuria and even mild ketonuria.

Honeymoon Period: Diabetes in children is often initially diagnosed in a medical emergency. After the crisis and after insulin therapy has been initiated there is a period of time known as the "honeymoon period" when the insulin requirement is low because the pancreas is still capable of producing some insulin. This period could last from 6 to 18 months. During this time insulin, in very small amounts, is given to help avoid problems that could occur when insulin is re-introduced.

Glucose Tolerance Test (GTT): Usually designated *OGTT* (oral). Comparison of glucose tolerance results with standard normal ranges requires standardized conditions. The individual should be ambulatory, otherwise healthy for two weeks prior to the test, receive a weight maintaining diet with a minimum of 150 grams of carbohydrate daily the three days prior to testing. After an overnight fast of 8 to 16 hours, a measured oral glucose load is given. The individual should rest 30 minutes before the test is given and remain seated during the test period. Water is permitted but smoking is not. Blood is taken before the test, one half, one, one and one half and two hours after glucose administration. There are special criteria used for children and during pregnancy. Diabetes Mellitus is indicated in non-pregnant adults when two or more OGTT are abnormal with plasma glucose values exceeding 200 mg/dL (11 mmol/L) at two hours and one other time.

Erroneous diagnosis of diabetes mellitus may occur in individuals for a variety of reasons such a drugs, hormones, stress, other clinical conditions and advanced age.

Caution is needed in the administration of OGTT because of the risk of severe hyperglycemia.

Fasting plasma glucose concentration exceeding normal levels by certain amounts on two or more occasions are also diagnostic.

Dietary essential amino acids — see proteins

Dietary fiber — see fiber

Dietary goals — see nutritional needs and food intake

Dietary guidelines — see nutritional needs and food intake

Dietary non-essential amino acids — see proteins

Dietitian — is an expert in nutrition who has met standards of education of The American Dietetic Association. An R.D. (registered dietitian) has demonstrated competency on a national examination. An L.D. (licensed dietitian) has met a state's requirement for licensure to practice.

Dietetic candies — see food terms

Diglycerides — see lipids

Disaccharides — see carbohydrates

Double sugars — see carbohydrates

Eating disorders:

Anorexia Nervosa: loss of appetite for food, not explainable by local disease; occurs most often in adolescence especially in girls but is also seen in males and young adult women. The patient exhibits extreme underweight due to self-denial in order to control his weight.

Bulimia: uncontrolled eating followed by induced vomiting; termed binge-purge syndrome. Bulimic patients are not usually underweight and may appear normal.

Diabetic Bulimics: may be a term that can be used to describe diabetics who binge and omit insulin to control their weight. The adverse effects on blood glucose levels of such a regime could be hazardous.

EFA, essential fatty acid — see lipids

Energy Terms:

Food Energy: is contained in molecules of carbohydrate, protein, lipids and alcohol. The metabolic oxidation of these molecules releases energy in the form of ATP (adenosine-tri-phosphate) and other high energy compounds that are used for metabolism and voluntary activity. The transfer of food energy to mechanical work occurs at a maximum efficiency of 25%. The remainder is used to maintain body temperature or is lost as heat.

calorie: a measure of heat. One calorie is the amount of energy required to raise the temperature of one gram of water through one degree Celsius.

Kilocalorie (kcal, also *Calorie* with capital C): the measure of energy used in nutrition. It is the amount of heat required to raise the temperature of one kilogram of water through one degree Celsius. Energy intake and expenditure are measured in kcals. The Calorie (kilocalorie) is 1,000 times larger than a calorie.

KiloJoule (kJ): Accepted as the international unit of energy measurement. One kiloJoule equals the energy required to lift one kilogram the height of one meter. The conversion is 1 kcal = 4.2 kJ. One megaJoule equals 1,000 kJ.

Metabolism: The sum of all of the physical and chemical processes that take place within the body that build and maintain the organism and the transformation by which energy is made available for use. Two fundamental processes are involved:

　　1. *Anabolism*: assimilation or building up processes and
　　2. *Catabolism*: disintegration or tearing down processes.

Basal Metabolism: Expressed as basal metabolic rate (BMR). Lowest level of energy expenditure determined under standardized resting conditions, 12-18 hours after eating and in controlled environmental conditions. Represents energy expended for maintenance of respiration, circulation, peristalsis, muscle tone, body temperature, glandular functions and other involuntary or unconscious functions of the body.

Resting Metabolism: Expressed as resting metabolic rate (RMR). Level of energy expenditure that represents all of the involuntary activities of the body as well as the after effect of exercise and of food. The RMR may be as much as 10% more than the BMR.

Enriched — see food terms

EPA, eicosapentaenoic acid — see lipids

"Equal" — see nutritive sweeteners

"Essentials of an Adequate Diet" — see nutrient needs and food intakes

Ethanol: For some people ethyl alcohol is the fourth class of energy nutrients. Alcohol provides 7 kcal per gram. Alcoholic beverages may supply other nutrients but in such small amounts as to be inconsequential. Excessive alcohol intake leads to increased formation of body lipids, especially triglycerides and cholesterol and decreased breakdown of fatty acids for energy. This decrease in fatty acid oxidation causes more glucose to be used for energy and a short term hypoglycemia may occur.

Euglycemia — see diabetes terms

Evaporated milk — see food terms

Evaporated skim milk — see food terms

Fasting blood glucose — see diabetes terms

Fats — see lipids

Fat substitutes and not fat substitutes:

"Nutrifat": New product based on carbohydrates and proteins formulated with edible oils. The ingredients are all GRAS (generally recognized as safe) substances so the product does not require FDA approval. It is not calorie-free but would certainly provide fewer kcals than if it were an all fat product.

"Simplesse": Product proposed by the Nutrasweet Company and currently under consideration by FDA. It is a combination of heat-coagulated milk protein and egg whites that have been treated to provide a feeling to the mouth similar to fat. It would provide 1-1/3 kcal per gram.

"No-cal Olestra": Product proposed by Proctor and Gamble and currently under consideration by FDA. It is a sucrose-polyester; fatty acids from a lipid such as soy oil, linked to 6, 7 or 8 esters of sucrose (instead of glyerol). It is calorie-free because it is not digested by humans or other animals.

Not a Fat Substitute: *Mineral Oil*: A refined petroleum product. It is not digested by humans or other animals. Use of mineral oil should be discouraged because it acts as a solvent for fat-soluble vitamins thus preventing their absorption because they are excreted with the mineral oil.

Fatty acids: see lipid terms

Fiber:

> *Dietary Fiber*: A term used to describe those components of plant cell walls that cannot be digested by human enzymes. They are primarily non-starch polysaccharides and can be classed as structural (cellulose and hemicellulose) or functional polysaccharides (pectins, gums, mucilages). Algae from seaweed is also in this group. Dietary fiber also includes *lignin, a non-carbohydrate* material of plants.

> *Crude Fiber*: A term denoting the material in plant foods which can be extracted by chemical treatment. It represents only a small fraction of dietary fiber and is not a useful term in nutrition.

> *Soluble Fiber*: Pectins, gums, mucilages, and some hemicelluloses. Sometimes called *"hemicellulosic"* or *"noncellulosic."*

> *Insoluble Fiber*: lignin, cellulose and some hemicelluloses. Sometimes called *"cellulosic."*

Filled milks and creams — see food terms

Food energy — see energy

Food fats — see lipids

Food Group Plans — see Nutrient Needs and Food Intake Terms

Food Terms:

> *Additives* (in food) — any substance not normally in a food which is either intentionally or accidently added.

> > *GRAS* (generally regarded as safe) list of food additives established by the FDA.

> *Enriched* — Addition of nutrients to a processed food, usually the nutrients present in the food before processing and lost or diminished in the processing.

> *Fortified* — Addition of nutrients to a food, often nutrients not present in the food originally.

> *Supplement* — A food to which nutrients have been added in amounts greater than 50% of the U.S. RDAs or any pill, powder or liquid that contains nutrients intended to supplement the diet.

Reduced Calorie — to be so labeled, a food must have at least one third fewer kcal than the expected energy value of that food and must have a nutritional label.

Low Calorie — to be labeled low calorie a food must have less than 40% of the energy value normally expected. The absolute kcal per serving must be stated.

Sodium Free — can be used on the label if the food contains less than 5 mg of sodium per serving.

Very Low Sodium — used if the product provides less than 35 mg per serving.

Reduced Sodium — a food using this statement on the label must be processed to reduce the sodium level by 75%.

Unsalted — the food was processed without the normally added salt.

"Health Food," "Natural Food," "Organic Food" — All are terms that have no legal definition. Popular meanings have been given to the terms, but the definitions are not universally accepted by those who are advocates.

Health Foods — a general term implying both natural and organic.

Natural Foods — foods altered as little as possible after harvest.

Organic Foods — foods fertilized with natural materials rather than formulated fertilizers, grown without the use of pesticides and processed without additives. (By chemical definition, all materials containing carbon are organic.)

"Junk Food": coined phrase used for foods providing a high proportion of energy in relation to the amounts of other essential nutrients or for foods low in nutrients but high in sugar, salt and fat.

Kosher: food selected and prepared according to Jewish dietary laws. The word is also used to describe foods allowed on diets of traditionally observant Jewish people.

Evaporated Milk: is canned whole fluid milk with about 60% of the water removed. It is fortified with 400 I.U. of Vitamin D per reconstituted quart. According to federal standards it must contain not less than 7.5% milk fat and not less than 25% total milk solids.

Evaporated Skim Milk: is canned skim fluid milk with about 60% of the water removed. It must contain not less than 20% milk solids. Vitamins A and D must be added to the product.

Sweetened Condensed Milk: has about 15% sugar added to whole fluid milk which is then concentrated to about one-third its initial volume. The finished product has a sucrose content of 42%. By federal standards it must have 28% total milk solids and 8% milk fat. Sweetened condensed milk has about three times more kcal than evaporated milk, about six times more sugar and about 25% more fat.

Filled Milks and Creams: have the natural butter fat replaced with vegetable fats. They contain the same calories as regular milk and cream.

Raw Milk: is milk in its natural state. Public Health authorities advocate pasteurization to destroy disease producing organisms. Milk for human consumption in interstate commerce must be pasteurized. The sale of raw milk is banned in 27 states.

Dietetic Candies: sweeteners in these products are often the sugar alcohols and may contain the same caloric content as regular candies. *Dietetic candy bars* frequently have a high fat content and are not recommended for diabetics. They are also sweetened with sugar alcohols. Sorbitol and mannitol are most often used.

Salad Dressings: no oil and reduced calorie salad dressings are available. The no oil dressings provide only an inconsequential amount of energy; whereas the reduced calorie dressings vary from a small amount of energy to the limit allowed by the FDA regulations for a reduced calorie food.

Cholesterol Altered: "Eggbeaters" is a low cholesterol egg substitute that is basically egg white. The name is a registered trademark.

Fortified — see food terms

Free fatty acids — see lipids, blood lipids

Fructose — see carbohydrates, nutritive sweeteners
Fruit and fruit juices — see nutritive sweeteners

Galactose — see carbohydrates
Glucagon — see diabetes terms
Glucose — see carbohydrates, nutritive sweeteners
Glucose tolerance test, GTT — see diabetes terms
Glycemic index — see diabetes terms
Glycerides — see lipids
Glycerol — see lipids
Glycolipids — see lipids
Glycosylated hemoglobin (HbA_{1c}) — see diabetes terms
Gums — see carbohydrates

"Health Foods" — see food terms
HDL, high density lipoproteins — see lipids, blood lipids
Hemicellulose — see carbohydrates, fiber
Hemicellulosic — see fiber
Hexoses — see carbohydrates
High biological value — see proteins
High fructose corn syrup — see nutritive sweeteners
Holistic approach — see questionable nutrition practices and approaches
Homeopathy — see questionable nutrition practices and approaches
Honey — see nutritive sweeteners
Honeymoon Period — see diabetes terms
Hydrogenation — see lipids
Hypercholesterolemia — see lipids, blood lipids
Hyperglycemia — see diabetes terms
Hyperlipidemia — see lipids, blood lipids
Hyperlipoproteinemia — see lipids, blood lipids
Hypertriglyceridemia — see lipids, blood lipids
Hypoglycemia — see diabetes terms

"Ideal Body Weight" — see body weight and wt/ht tables
Insoluble fiber — see fiber
Insulin — see diabetes terms
Iridology — see questionable nutrition practices and approaches

"Junk Food" — see food terms

Ketone bodies — see diabetes terms
Ketosis, ketoacidosis — see diabetes terms
Kilocalorie — see energy
KiloJoule — see energy
Kosher — see food terms

Lacto-ovo-vegetarian — see alternate eating patterns
Lactose — see carbohydrates
Lactose Intolerance: Intolerance to lactose, the disaccharide sugar
    of milk, is primarily due to a total or partial lack of the enzyme
    lactase (in the small intestine) that splits lactose into glucose and
    galactose. Symptoms of lactose intolerance include abdominal
    cramps, diarrhea and flatulence.
LDL, low density lipoproteins — see lipids, blood lipids
Lignin — see fiber
Linoleic acid — see lipids
Linolenic acid — see lipids
Lipids: Any one of a group of fats or fat-like substances that are
    characterized by their relative insolubility in water. One of the
    three major classes of energy nutrients and the major stored en-
    ergy component of the body. All lipids contribute 9 kcal per
    gram. Dietary lipids are primarily *triglycerides* in which three
    fatty acids, the building blocks of lipids, are combined with the
    alcohol *glycerol*. These are also called *neutral fats, triacylglyc-*
    erols or *glycerides*.
        Diglycerides and *monoglycerides* (two fatty acids or one fatty
        acid attached to glycerol) are also found in nature. (These
        lipids are good emulsifying agents so their names appear on
        ingredient listings of food labels.) In addition to triglyc-
        erides, fatty acids are the building blocks of other lipids, the
        phosphoglycerides, glycolipids, cholesterol esters and some
        waxes. More than 70 different fatty acids have been identi-
        fied. They differ in the length of the carbon atom chains, the
        degree of saturation (number of double bonds) and in the
        placement of the double bonds between the carbon atoms.
        Fatty acids occurring in higher plants and animals generally

have an even number of carbon atoms that occur as chains of from 4 to 22 carbon atoms, with 16-18 carbon chains the most common. The fatty acids can be *saturated* (have no double bonds), *monounsaturated* (have one double bond) or be *polyunsaturated* (have 2 or more double bonds between the carbon atoms).

Fats/Oils: Each lipid is composed of a variety of fatty acids and the physical characteristics (solid or liquid) of lipids in food will be determined by the total effect of all the fatty acids present. Generally fatty acids with short carbon chains or highly unsaturated are liquid at room temperature (oils); whereas lipids with long chains or saturated fatty acids are solid at room temperature (fats). However, just because a lipid is a liquid at room temperature, does not always mean that it contains many polyunsaturated fatty acids.

Essential Fatty Acid (EFA): The human body can synthesize all the fatty acids needed by the body except for one. End products from carbohydrate, protein and lipid breakdown are used for the synthesis of fatty acids. The *EFA* is called *linoleic* acid. It is an 18 carbon chain with two double bonds, designated as 9,12-octadecadienoic acid or 18:2 omega 6, or 18:2 N-6. It belongs to the class of omega 6 fatty acids. Other than linoleic acid, humans have no need for dietary fats except as a source of energy or as the carrier for fat soluble vitamins.

Polyunsaturated Fatty Acids (PUFA): There are two major groups of PUFA: (1) is the *omega 6* or N-6 series with linoleic acid (18:2, N-6) from vegetable sources as the major supplier; (2) the second class is the *omega three* series or N-3 series with linolenic acid (18:3, N-3) as the major source. Linolenic acid is found in low concentration in leafy plant tissues and in soybean oil. In the body linoleic is elongated to arachidonic acid (20:4, N-6) eicosatetraenoic acid, but the conversion of linolenic acid (octadecatrienoic acid, 18:3, N-3) to its counterpart *eicosapentaenoic acid* (EPA), 20:5, N-3) does not occur to any great extent. Considerable research is being done at the present time on the physiological effects of the omega three fatty acids. Two that are receiving the most attention are *EPA*, eicosapentaenoic acid, 20:5, N-3, and *DHA*, docosahexaenoic acid, 22:6, N-3. These polyunsaturated fatty acids are found primarily in marine animal lipids.

Sterols: The cholesterol esters are the best known lipids in this class. Cholesterol is found only in animal tissues and synthesized by the human body. One form (7-dehydro cholesterol) is converted to active vitamin D in the body with sunlight. The greater part of the cholesterol in the body arises from synthesis with dietary cholesterol contributing a smaller portion. Cholesterol is the parent compound of all the steroids synthesized in the body.

Blood Lipids: Lipids are not soluble in water so in order for them to be transported through the blood (an aqueous medium) they are combined with protein to form lipoprotein complexes. Apart from *free fatty acids* (bound to the protein albumin) which account for only a small percent of the total blood lipids, four major fractions of blood lipids have been characterized. These are: (1) *chylomicrons* which arise from the intestines, (2) *VLDL*, very low density lipoproteins which come from the intestines and liver, (3) *LDL*, low density lipoproteins, from VLDL and chylomicrons, and (4) *HDL*, high density lipoproteins from mainly the liver and intestines. Free fatty acids arise predominantly from adipose tissue. All four of the fractions contain triglycerides, phospholipids, and cholesterol esters in addition to protein, but in differing amounts. For example, chylomicrons contain the most total lipid, the most triglycerides and the least protein; whereas the HDL fraction contains the most protein and the least triglyceride. Both the LDL and the HDL fractions contain more free and esterified cholesterol than the other fractions with the LDLs normally carrying the greater amount.

Hyperlipidemia: Excess of any lipid constituent of the blood, e.g.:

Hypercholesterolemia: Elevated concentration of cholesterol in the blood.

Hypertriglyceridemia: Elevated level of triglycerides in the blood.

Hyperlipoproteinemia: The excess of any one of the lipoprotein fractions in the blood and usually accompanied by hyperlipidemia. Measurement of the various lipoprotein fractions of the blood by electrophoresis is the basis for the classification of the hyperlipoproteinemias into types based upon the fraction(s) which show increased concentration. These types have been designated as I, IIA, IIB, III, IV, and V. Type IIB and type IV are most often seen in diabetics, especially NIDDM. In type IIB, VLDL and LDL fractions are elevated resulting in increased levels of cholesterol and triglycerides. In type IV, VLDL levels are increased resulting in increased levels of triglycerides and either elevated or normal levels of cholesterol.

Food Fats vs. Blood Lipids:

Food Fats are described as solid or liquid, animal or vegetable, saturated or unsaturated and termed shortenings, spreads or oils. Cholesterol is a separate type of food fat. Regardless of the type or characteristic of food fats, all yield 9 kcal/g.

Blood Lipids are the product of synthesis by the body from the monosaccharides, amino acids, fatty acids, alcohol and other materials furnished as products of digestion. The only exception to this is the blood lipid fraction, the chylomicrons, which represent the transport of lipids from the digestive tract to the liver. There is an interconversion of food stuffs in the body so that carbohydrates can become fatty acids, amino acids or another material or be used as energy. The same is true of amino acids, fatty acids and cholesterol. Elevated triglycerides in the blood are often the result of too much dietary carbohydrate and/or an excess intake of kcals, or they could be from a metabolic malfunction of undetermined origin rather than from excess dietary intake.

Hydrogenation: Term used with food fats. Hydrogen is introduced into the carbon chain of fatty acids in a food fat and is attached at the carbon atoms near the double bonds. This chemical process converts a liquid (oil) with unsaturated carbon atoms into a more solid (fat) with additional saturated carbon atoms.

P/S Ratio: Term used with food fats. It is the ratio of polyunsaturated to saturated fats in the diet. Although some
ratios have been suggested, the current trend is to follow
the "Dietary Goals."
Low calorie — see food terms

Maltose — see carbohydrates
Mannitol — see carbohydrates, nutritive sweeteners
Maple syrup — see nutritive sweeteners
MegaJoule — see energy
Metabolism — see energy
Metric and English Systems of Weights and Measures

Metric	English
28.35 g (grams)	1 oz (ounce)
453.59 g	1 lb (pound)
1 kg (kilogram) (10^3)	2.2 lb
29.57 ml (milliliters) (10^{-3})	1 fluid ounce
236.58 ml	8 fluid oz (1 cup)
473.17 ml	16 fluid oz (1 pint)
946.33 ml	32 fluid oz (1 quart)
1 L (liter)	33.81 fluid oz
2.54 cm (centimeters) (10^{-2})	1 inch
30.48 cm	1 foot (12 in)
0.9144 m (meters)	1 yard (36 in)
1 m (meter)	39.37 in

Milk, evaporated, skim, sweetened condensed, and raw — see food
terms
Mineral oil — see not a fat substitute
Molasses — see nutritive sweeteners
Mole — see SI units
Monoglycerides — see lipids
Monosaccharides — see carbohydrates
Monounsaturated — see lipids
Mucilages — see carbohydrates, fiber

"National Food Guide" — see nutrient needs and food intake

"National Wartime Nutrition Guide" — see nutrient needs and food intake

Natural foods — see food terms

Naturopathy — see questionable nutrition practices and approaches

Neutral fats — see lipids

"No-cal-olestra" — see fat substitutes

Noncellulosic — see fiber

Non-Nutritive Sweeteners

> *Cyclamate*: a sweetener approximately 30 times sweeter than sucrose was discovered in 1937 and marketed as cyclamic acid, calcium cyclamate and sodium cyclamate. It was banned by the FDA in 1969 because it was implicated as a cancer causing agent in rats. Further research failed to prove the carcinogenicity of cyclamate but FDA rejected a 1980 petition for approval. Reapproval was sought and is expected.

> *Saccharin* is the only non-nutritive sweetener available on the market at the present time. It is an organic compound about 300 times as sweet as sucrose, is colorless, odorless and water soluble.

> Other non-nutritive sweeteners *in* various stages of *development* are:

> *Neohesperidin*: from rind of oranges and grapefruit, can be converted to a material which has a sweetening power 1000-2000 times that of sugar — not approved by FDA.

> *Narigin*: from grapefruit rinds, has a sweetening power of about 1500 times that of sugar — not approved. Other chemicals are being tested and there may be new non-nutritive sweeteners available in the future.

Non-structural polysaccharides — see carbohydrates

Normoglycemia — see diabetes terms

"Nutrasweet" — see nutritive sweeteners

Nutrient Needs and Food Intake Terms:

> *RDAs*: Recommended Daily Dietary Allowances established by the Food and Nutrition Board of the National Research Council National Academy of Sciences. The RDAs are levels of intake of essential nutrients considered to be adequate to meet the known nutritional needs of almost all healthy

persons. Levels established are for 19 nutrients plus energy for both sexes in various age groups.

U.S. RDAs: Established for labeling of foods by the FDA (Food and Drug Administration) in 1973. The 1968 National Research Council RDAs were used as a basis, and the FDA established the U.S. RDAs listing the highest value (except for pregnant and lactating women) for each nutrient at any age level except for calcium and phosphorus. They also included values for biotin, pantothenic acid, copper and zinc (not included in RDAs) in addition to the 17 nutrients plus energy of the RDAs. The FDA also established 50% and 150% levels of the nutrients; 50% being half, 150% 1 1/2 times the U.S. RDA figures. For formulated or fabricated food containing up to 50%, nutritional labeling is adequate. If this product contains more than 50% of the U.S. RDA for a nutrient, it is considered a dietary supplement just as an "over-the-counter" vitamin or multi supplement. If the formulated or fabricated product provides a nutrient at levels over 150% of the U.S. RDA, the product is considered a drug.

Dietary Guidelines: Established for the purpose of identifying kinds of foods (and amounts) needed daily to meet the nutritional needs known at the time.

First Guide in 1917 by USDA had five food groups: flesh foods, starchy foods, fat foods, watery fruits and vegetables, and sweets. Revision in 1933 contained 12 food groups and were presented at three different cost levels.

"National Wartime Nutrition Guide" and its revision the *"National Food Guide"* were published by USDA shortly after the first RDAs were set forth (1941). The National Food Guide became known as the *"Basic Seven Food Group Guide."*

The National Food Guide served as the basis for the *"Basic Four Food Group Guide"* which was published by USDA in a 1958 publication "Food for Fitness—A Daily Food Guide." This grouping put the fruit and vegetable groups together and eliminated the butter and margarine thus condensing the seven groups to four. It was also termed *"Essentials of an Adequate Diet."* No new daily guide has been established since that time although the USDA in 1979 issued a publication entitled *"Hassle Free Guide to a Better Diet"* which included five groups. The fifth group—fats, sweets and alcohol, but no servings were recommended. The first edition of the *"Dietary Goals"* by the Senate Select Committee on Nutrition and Human Needs was published in 1977 and was followed by a joint publication with the USDA—*"Nutrition and Your Health, Dietary Guidelines for Americans"* in 1980. These guidelines were broad suggestions rather than specific recommendations for kinds and amounts of food. The Dietary Goals and The Basic Four food plan are not exactly compatible because one of the underlying premises of the dietary goals was disease prevention which was not a consideration for the development of the four food group plan.

"Nutrifat"—see fat substitutes

"Nutrition and Your Health, Dietary Guidelines for Americans"— see nutrient needs and food intake

Nutritionist—is not a legal term. Anyone can call her/himself a nutritionist (See dietitian).

Nutritive Sweeteners: Any number of compounds with a sweet taste and which produces energy in the body.

  Sucrose: Table sugar. It is granulated sugar from sugar cane or sugar beets. It is also available in cube or powdered form or as brown sugar. It provides 4 kcal per gram.

  Fructose: A monosaccharide, sweeter than sucrose. It is found free in fruit, fruit juices, vegetables, honey and other foods. It is commercially available in the free form. It provides 4 kcal per gram.

  Glucose: Also called dextrose. It is a monosaccharide and along with fructose is an end product of sucrose digestion. It is also an end product of the digestion of the disaccharides maltose and lactose. It occurs free in fruit and fruit juices, honey and other fruits and vegetables. It is available commercially in the pure form. It provides 4 kcal per gram.

  Raw Sugar: Is unrefined cane or beet sugar containing about

96% pure sucrose. Its sale is banned by the Food and Drug Administration because it is highly contaminated.

Turbinado Sugar: Is the product resulting from treatment of raw sugar (separated and washed with steam). Part of its molasses is removed, but it keeps a light brown color. It is 99% sucrose, but the water content will vary. The products are *not* labeled raw sugar; however, a "Sugar in the Raw" label appears acceptable. It provides 4 kcal per gram.

Corn Syrup: Is made from corn starch, the amount of glucose present is dependent on the type of manufacturing process used. It also contains maltose which is not as sweet as the other sugars. It provides 4 kcal per gram.

High Fructose Corn Syrup: Is commercially produced from high glucose corn syrup and can contain as much as 90% fructose. It is very sweet since fructose is the sweetest of the sugars. It provides 4 kcal per gram.

Molasses: Is the residue remaining after sucrose crystals have been removed from the concentrated beet or cane juices. It contains sucrose, glucose and fructose.

Sorghum: Is the syrup of sorghum cane. It is similar in composition to molasses.

Maple Syrup: Is obtained from the sap of the sugar maple trees. After concentration, the syrup contains about 65% sugar, most of which is sucrose.

Honey: Produced by honey bees from the nectar of flowers. It contains more fructose than other sugar syrups except for high fructose corn syrup, and therefore, is sweeter than other syrups. Commercial honey is cleaned before being placed on the market. The process involves heating the honey to 140° F., held at that temperature for 30 minutes and then strained. This heat treatment is not severe enough to kill all the Clostridium botulinum which can be present. The small amounts are probably not a problem for adults but may be hazardous to infants and young children.

Aspartame: Is a compound composed of two amino acids (aspartic acid and phenylalanine) which when combined have a very sweet taste. Although aspartame is not a carbohydrate, it is considered a nutritive sweetener because the two amino acids are metabolized in the body as other amino acids and yield 4 kcal per gram. However, aspartame is about 200 times sweeter than table sugar so only a small amount is needed. Aspartame is marketed under the trade names Equal™ and Nutrasweet.™ One packet of Equal with 4 kcal is equivalent in sweetening ability to two teaspoons of table sugar.

Acesulfame-K (Sunette™) is derived from acetoacetic acid. The product is marketed as "Sweet One" and contains dextrose and cream of tartar in addition to acesulfame-K. Each packet which is equivalent in sweetening to two teaspoons of sucrose contains 4 kcals. Sweet One™ has the advantage of heat and pH stability and can be substituted for 1/2 of the sugar in baked products.

Sugar Alcohols: Sorbitol, mannitol and xylitol, the main sugar alcohols, are almost as sweet as glucose. Sorbitol is the most frequently used. It is poorly absorbed and may cause abdominal distress, but what is absorbed is converted to fructose in the liver and is gradually converted to glucose, contributing to the blood glucose level. The sugar alcohols provide 4 kcal per gram.

Fruit and Fruit Juices: Are dilute sugar solutions containing primarily fructose, glucose and sucrose. In contrast to the other nutritive sweeteners, fruits and fruit juices provide other nutrients in addition to energy.

Obesity — see body weight and wt/ht terms
Oils — see lipids
Oligosaccharides — see carbohydrates
Omega-3 fatty acids — see lipids
Omega-6 fatty acids — see lipids
Oral glucose tolerance test, OGTT — see diabetes terms
"Organic foods" — see food terms
Overweight — see body weight terms

Pectins — see carbohydrates, fiber
Phosphoglycerides — see lipids
Polysaccharides — see carbohydrates

Polyunsaturated fatty acids — see lipids

Postprandial — see diabetes terms

Preprandial — see diabetes terms

Protein quality — see proteins

Proteins: One of the three main classes of energy nutrients. They are large organic materials whose basic units are amino acids. Amino acids are characterized by the presence of nitrogen as an amino group ($-NH_2$). *Simple proteins* are composed of amino acids only whereas *complex proteins* contain non-protein material in addition to amino acids. Proteins can be further classified on the basis of (1) solubility, (2) overall shape, (3) function and (4) physical properties. Proteins are essential in the diet for supplying amino acids for the synthesis of almost all body tissues and fluids. All food proteins supply 4 kcal per gram.

> *Dietary Essential and Non-essential Amino Acids*: Amino acids are termed either dietary essentials or non-essentials. The *dietary essential amino acids* are those that cannot be synthesized by the human body and therefore must be provided preformed from food. The *dietary non-essential amino acids* are those that the human body can synthesize when amino nitrogen is present. Of the 20 commonly known amino acids, 9 are dietary essentials, but all 20 of the amino acids are necessary for synthesis of body proteins.

> *Protein Quality*: The quality of food proteins in terms of usefulness to the body is described as *biological value*. A protein food is of *high biological value* when it is digestible, contains all the dietary essential amino acids in amounts and proportions needed by man and furnishes sufficient amino nitrogen for synthesis of other amino acids to form proteins in the body.

> *Complimentary Proteins*: Two or more foods whose proteins are of low biological value that when ingested together, the combined amino acids will be complimentary and meet the body's need.

P/S, polyunsaturated to saturated fatty acid ratio — see lipids

Questionable Nutrition Practices and Approaches: Currently advocated by groups antagonistic toward accepted medical practice.

Autointoxication: A theory promoting the idea that chronic poisoning of the body occurs as a result of intestinal stasis which allows intestinal contents to putrify and form toxins which are absorbed, poisoning the body. No such toxins have ever been found.

Chelation Therapy: Promoted to restore atherosclerotic arteries to normal by using a chelating agent (frequently the synthetic amino acid EDTA) to remove calcium deposits. EDTA is injected into the veins. No scientific evidence supports this theory.

Colonic Irrigation: Supposed to irrigate the colon and remove undesirable wastes from the body. A rubber tube is inserted into the rectum for 20 to 30 inches and warm water up to 20 gallons is pumped in and out. Other substances may be added to the water such as herbs or coffee. This is a hazardous practice and has caused fatal infections.

Cytoxic Testing: Used to supposedly diagnose allergies by examining an individual's white blood cells under a microscope and checking the reaction of the cells to dried food extracts. White blood cells do not provide a reliable measure for determining allergies.

Holistic Approach: A term used by orthodox practitioners meaning the treatment of the whole person. The term when used by unscientific proponents appears to involve cosmic philosophy, unproven products and services, and antagonism toward accepted medical practices.

Homeopathy: Theory based on the premise that the more dilute a remedy the more powerful is its curative effect. This has no scientific or medical basis.

Iridology: A diagnostic system based upon the idea that each area of the body is represented by a certain area in the iris of the eye. Imbalances, determined by so-called practitioners of this theory, are treated with vitamins, minerals, herbs, etc. There is no scientific basis for diagnosis by the eyes.

Naturopathy: The basis for this practice is that the cause of disease is a violation of nature's laws and that diseases are the body's effort to purify itself. The cure for disease is to increase the patient's vital forces by ridding the body of toxins. This is accomplished with "natural food" diets, supplements, herbs, cell salts, etc. plus physical manipulations such as massage, colonic enemas, etc. This practice has no scientific basis.

Raw milk — see food terms
Raw sugar — see nutritive sweeteners
Rebound hyperglycemia — see diabetes terms
Recommended Daily Dietary Allowances, RDAs — see nutrient needs and food intake
Recommended weights in relation to heights — see body weight and wt/ht tables
Reduced calorie — see food terms
Resting metabolism — see energy

Salad dressings — see food terms
Saccharin — see non-nutritive sweeteners
Saturated fatty acids — see lipids
Simple proteins — see proteins
"Simplesse" — see fat substitutes
Simple sugar — see carbohydrates
"SI Units" is the abbreviation for *le Système international d'Unités* used to report clinical laboratory data. These SI units are replacing the various units that have been used to report laboratory information in the U.S. In the SI, the laboratory results are reported in units related to the amount of a substance. These are expressed in terms of moles per liter. The major changes affecting the reporting of clinical data are: (1) the referencing of all values to the liter and (2) the amount of substance is described in moles or their subunits rather than in mass terms as grams or milligrams.

   The SI has seven base units from which other units are derived. These are listed below with the property or physical quantity to which they refer and their official symbol:

Physical Quantity	Base Unit	SI Symbol
Length	meter	m
Mass	kilogram	kg

Time	second	s
Amount of Substance	mole	mol
Thermodynamic Temperature	Kelvin	K
Electric Current	Ampere	A
Luminous Intensity	candela	cd

The system uses a series of prefixes to the base unit to form decimal multiples and submultiples. The preferred intervals are 10^3 or 10^{-3} but some intervals less than these are occasionally used. The following table shows the preferred multiples and submultiples and the exceptions along with the symbol for each prefix.

```
    Factor              Prefix              Symbol
    10¹⁸                 exa                   E
    10¹⁵                peta                   P
    10¹²                tera                   T
    10⁹                 giga                   G
    10⁶                 mega                   M
    10³                 kilo                   k
  :-------------------------------------------------:
  :  10²               hecto                  h    :
  :  10¹               deka                   da   :
  :  10⁻¹              deci                   d    :
  :  10⁻²              centi                  c    :
  :-------------------------------------------------:
    10⁻³               milli                  m
    10⁻⁶               micro                  u
    10⁻⁹               nano                   n
    10⁻¹²              pico                   p
    10⁻¹⁵              fento                  f
    10⁻¹⁸              atto                   a
  Boxed factors are exceptions

  A mole is a quantity of a chemical compound whose
    weight in grams equals its molecular weight.   Thus
    one mole of water (H₂O) is 18.0154 g.
    Hydrogen atomic weight = 1.0080
    H₂                      = 2.0160
    Oxygen atomic weight    =15.9994
    therefore
                    2.0160
                  +15.9994
                   18.0154 is the formula mass of H₂O
                        and is one mol
  Tables are available giving the conversion factors for
  changing present reference intervals to the SI Reference
  intervals.
```

Example:

	Present Reference Interval	Present Unit	Conversion Factor	SI Reference Interval	SI Unit Symbol
Glucose (P) fasting	70-110	mg/dL	0.05551	3.9-6.1	mmol/L
	70 x 0.05551 = 3.9				
	110 x 0.05551 = 6.1				
Cholesterol(P)	200	mg/dL	0.02586	5.20	mmol/L
Potassium(S)	3.5-5	mEq/L	1.00	3.5-5	mmol/L
Fructose(P)	<10	mg/dL	0.05551	<0.6	mmol/L
Insulin(P)(S)	5-20	uU/mL	7.175	35-145	pmol/L
Calcium ion(S)	2.0-2.3	mEq/L	0.500	1.0-1.15	mmol/L
Sodium ion(S)	135-147	mEq/L	1.0	135-147	mmol/L

(P) plasma
(S) serum

Sodium—is an element essential to humans. The most common source is table salt where it is combined with chlorine as NaCl. It is also found naturally in many foods or furnished by drinking water or added to foods in processing. One teaspoon of NaCl weighs 6 grams and contains 2,300 mg of sodium. The human body requires only a small amount of sodium per day (estimated at 115-300 mg). The 1989 RDAs established a minimum daily requirement of 500 mg of sodium. Diet orders given in milliequivalents can be converted to milligrams as 23 mEq = 1 mg Na. In SI units 1 mEq Na = 1 mmol.

Sodium free, very low, reduced—see food terms

Soluble fiber—see fiber

Somogyi effect—see diabetes terms

Sorbitol—see carbohydrates, nutritive sweeteners

Sorghum—see nutritive sweeteners

Starch—see carbohydrates

Sterols—see lipids

Structural polysaccharides—see carbohydrates, fiber

Sucrose—see carbohydrates, nutritive sweeteners

Sugar alcohols—see carbohydrates, nutritive sweeteners

Sugars—see carbohydrates, nutritive sweeteners

Supplements—see food terms

Table sugar—see carbohydrates, nutritive sweeteners

Triacylglycerols—see lipids

Triglycerides — see lipids
Turbinado sugar — see food items

Underweight — see body weight terms
Unsalted — see food terms
U.S RDAs — see nutritional needs, food intake

Vegan — see alternate eating patterns
Vegetarian — see alternate eating patterns
VLDL, very low density lipoproteins — see lipids, blood lipids

Waxes — see lipids

Xylitol — see carbohydrates, nutritive sweeteners

Index

sample menus, 207-211
Honey, 122
Hospitalized patients, diabetic
  with cancer, 95-96
  carbohydrate requirements, 67,81,
    82
  diet prescription, 67,80
  discharge diets, 80,83
  drug-nutrient interactions, 96-99
  elderly, 66-68,69-70
  electrolyte balance-imbalance,
    91-94
  energy requirements, 81,82
    energy prescription, 79
  Exchange List Patterns, 80
  fat-controlled diets, 89-90
  fat requirements, 81,82
  fiber requirements, 81,82
  with gastrointestinal disorders,
    94-95
  protein requirements, 81,82
  with renal failure, 90-91,116
  sodium requirements, 81,82
  special diets, 84-89
  weight loss, 67
Hunger, 102
Hyperglycemia
  in adolescents, 44
  in children, 37
Hyperlipoproteinemia, 89,90
Hypoglycemia
  in children, 37,40
  dietary treatment, 47-49
  during pregnancy, 51
  weight control and, 101,102
Hypolipoproteinemia, 117

Iditarod dog race, energy use
    estimation method for, 47,48
Infants, diabetic, 33-35
  growth grids, 33
  infant formulas, 33-34
  insulin adjustment, 33
  Recommended Daily Allowances,
    35
  solid foods, 33-35

Insulin
  children's requirements, 35
  blood glucose effects, 70
  for gestational diabetes, 53
  infants' requirements, 33
  pregnant women's requirements,
    50
  protein-by-weight ratio, 119-120
  weight control and, 101-102
Iron, 34,52
Iron supplement, 61
Irritants, gastric, 94

Jewish food patterns, 69,71,73-74

Kashruth, 73
Kentucky Diabetes Foundation, 29
Ketosis
  appetite effects, 103
  patient-induced, 101-102
  during pregnancy, 51
Kilocalorie, 126
  alcohol content, 116
  Four Food Groups content,
    117-118
  liquid diet content, 86-89
  in renal failure, 91
Kosher food, 71,73-74

Lactation
  fiber intake during, 53
  Recommended Daily Allowances
    during, 82
  sample menus, 203-205
Lactose, in renal failure, 91
Lactose deficiency, 36,94
Liquid diet, 84-89
  high-sucrose, 94,115
  for weight loss, 109
Low-calorie diet, 102-103
Low-cholesterol diet, 90,115
Low-fat diet, 90
Low-protein diet, 91
Low-residue diet, 95